AROMATHERAPY
Therapy Basics

second edition

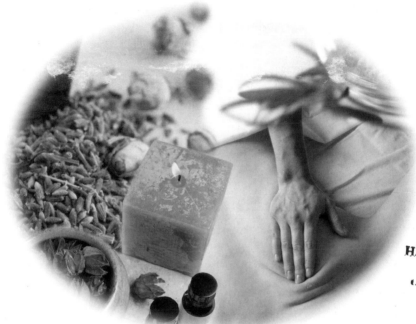

HELEN McGUINNESS

Hodder Arnold

A MEMBER OF THE HODDER HEADLINE GROUP

Orders: please contact Bookpoint Ltd, 130 Milton Park, Abingdon, Oxon OX14 4SB. Telephone: (44) 01235 827720.
Fax: (44) 01235 400454. Lines are open from 9.00 – 5.00, Monday to Saturday, with a 24 hour message answering service.
You can also order through our website: www.hoddereducation.co.uk

British Library Cataloguing in Publication Data
A catalogue record for this title is available from the British Library

ISBN 978 0 340 87680 0

First edition published 1997
This edition published 2003

Impression number   10 9 8 7 6 5
Year   2010   2009   2008   2007

Cover photo from Photodisc
Typeset by Fakenham Photosetting Ltd, Fakenham, Norfolk.
Printed in India for Hodder Arnold, an imprint of Hodder Education, a division of Hodder Headline, an Hachette Livre UK Company,
338 Euston Road, London NW1 3BH by Replika Press Pvt. Ltd.

Contents

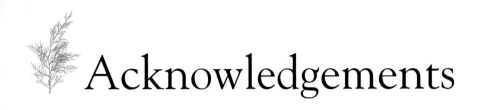

Acknowledgements

I would like to extend my thanks to my father, Roy, for his great skill in producing the illustrations for this book, and to my mother, Valerie, for her patience in checking the text for grammar, and especially for her encouragement. My thanks also goes to my husband, Mark, who has provided considerable help, love and support throughout the development of this book.

My grateful thanks also extends to the following people:

Deirdre Moynihan and Stephanie Mealey of AVCS for their technical help in checking the accuracy of the text and for their valued contributions; John Marks for his technical help with the aroma chemistry chapter; Chris Ockendon of New Horizon Aromatics for his valued contributions to the text; Berni Hephrun of Butterbur and Sage for supplying information regarding the quality of essential oils; Alan Harris, the secretary of the ATC for providing me with valuable information. I would also like to express my gratitude to the AOC (Aromatherapy Organisations Council) for their valuable information on research; to Pamela Trodd and Karen Harrisson for their valued feedback on the first edition of this book. My sincere thanks to Nicole Cameron (a student at the Holistic Training Centre) for kindly granting use of her case study. Finally, thanks are due to all my students at the Holistic Training Centre, Southampton, for their support and encouragement in the development of the book and for their valued contributions.

For the reproduction of photographs the publisher would like to thank the following:
Photos 1, 3, 4, 6, 7, 8, 9, 10, 12, 13, 14, 15, 16, 17, 18, 19, 20, 21, 22, 23, 25, 28, 30, 31, 32, 34, 35, 36 courtesy of The Holt Studios Photographic Library; Photos 2, 5 , 11, 26, 26, 27, 29, 33, 37, 38 courtesy of The Garden Picture Library; and Photos 39, 40, 41 courtesy of Getty Images.

Introduction

Aromatherapy has grown in popularity over the past ten years to become recognised as a complementary therapy, and for those interested in holistic health care, it offers a very rewarding career.

This workbook is intended for those undertaking a professional course of training in aromatherapy or for qualified aromatherapists who want to update and extend their knowledge of the subject. It meets the underpinning knowledge requirements of the NVQ Level III in Aromatherapy Massage, but also covers the knowledge requirements of more traditional diploma courses.

The material contained within the book has been designed to be interactive. Each chapter has tasks and self-assessment questions to complete, in order to assess overall understanding of the individual subject areas.

As well as providing a comprehensive knowledge of aromatherapy, the aim of the workbook is to help candidates to generate portfolio evidence of underpinning knowledge for their NVQ qualification.

CHAPTER 1

Introduction to Aromatherapy

> *Aromatherapy is the art of using essential oils to help restore balance in the body, and is a form of natural healing that is more than 8,000 years old. Today it represents one of the fastest growing complementary therapies in the UK.*

✳ A competent aromatherapist needs to be able to understand aromatherapy as a holistic therapy, in order to apply suitable treatments, and give accurate advice and guidance to clients.

Objectives

By the end of this chapter you will be able to relate the following knowledge to your practical work carried out as an aromatherapist:

✳ how aromatherapy has developed

✳ uses of aromatherapy.

Aromatherapy can be defined as the systematic use of essential oils in holistic treatments to help improve physical and emotional well-being.

Aromatherapy is a truly holistic therapy, as it aims to treat the whole person by taking account not only of their physical state but also their emotions, which can have a profound effect on general well-being. It works on the principle that the most effective way to promote health and prevent illness is to strengthen the body's immune system; in so doing, it helps to restore the harmony between mind and body.

The primary form of aromatherapy applications involves using essential oils in the following ways:

✳ topically to the skin via massage, diluted in a carrier oil

✳ inhalations

✳ compresses

✳ aromatic baths.

An essential oil is the highly concentrated volatile substance obtained from various parts of the aromatic plant.

Disillusionment with orthodox medicine has caused many people to turn to the natural remedies that have been part of our folklore for many thousands of years.

The History of Aromatherapy

The history of the application of essential oils to the human body goes back to at least 2000 BC. Records in the Bible show the use of plants and their aromatic oils both for the treatment of illness and for religous purposes.

The first evidence of the wide-ranging use of aromatic oils comes from Ancient Egypt – Egyptians extracted oils by a method of infusion, and used them as cosmetics. One of the most famous Egyptian aromatic formulas was a mixture of 16 aromatic substances called 'kyphi', which was later used as a perfume by the Greeks and Romans. One of the earliest uses of aromatic oils by the Egyptians was incense for religious purposes and for embalming the dead to delay decomposition of bodies.

The ancient Greeks and Romans acquired much of their knowledge regarding the use of aromatic oils from the Egyptians. The Greek, Herodotus, was the first person to record the method of distillation of turpentine, around 425 BC.

The Greeks and Romans used aromatic oils for aromatic massages and in daily baths. They discovered that the odour of certain plants and flowers was stimulating and invigorating, while others were sedative and relaxing. The Greek soldiers also carried essential oils such as myrrh into battle with them for the treatment of wounds. Hippocrates, a Greek physician, wrote about a vast range of medicinal plants, and claimed that the best way to achieve good health was to have an aromatic bath and scented massage every day!

The writings of Hippocrates and others were translated into Arabic languages; after the fall of Rome and the advent of Christianity, surviving Roman physicians fled to Constantinople, taking their books and knowledge with them.

The most famous Arab physician was Avicenna, who reputedly wrote over 100 books describing over 800 plants and their effects on the body. However, his most important act in terms of aromatherapy is being credited with inventing the refrigerated coil, a development of the more primitive form of distillation, which he used to produce pure oils and aromatic waters.

The earliest written record of the use of aromatic oils in England was in the 13th century. From 1470–1670, the invention and development of printing across Europe resulted in the publication of many herbals or books that included recipes for making essential oils. It is a known fact that people who used aromatic oils were the only ones to survive the Plague that struck Europe during these centuries, due to the fact that the vast majority of essential oils have antiseptic properties.

The knowledge of the *medicinal* properties of plants was later reinforced by Nicholas Culpeper, a celebrated herbalist who wrote a book of herbs in 1652, which contained the medicinal properties of hundreds of plants.

Modern developments

The *scientific* study of the therapeutic properties of essential oils was commenced by the French cosmetic chemist, Renee Gattefosse, in the 1920s. He discovered through burning his arm while making fragrances in his laboratory, that the essential oil of lavender was exceptionally healing to the skin, and left no scarring. This discovery led him to undertake a great deal of research into the medicinal uses of essential oils, and his work revealed that it is possible for essential oils to penetrate the skin and be carried in the blood and lymphatic system to the organs.

Other French doctors and scientists continued his work and helped to validate the status of essential oils as scientific substances. Most notably, Dr Jean Valnet used essential oils to treat severe burns and battle injuries, in the absence of medical supplies. His book *Aromatherapie* (translated as *The Practice of Aromatherapy*) confirms the findings of Gattefosse, and has become an established textbook among serious aromatherapy practitioners.

Despite this, however, herbal medicine and aromatic remedies lost credibility with the growth of modern synthetic drug industry. By the middle of the 20th century, the role of essential oils was reduced to being employed in the perfumes, cosmetic and food industries.

Aromatherapy in Britain

The term 'aromatherapy' was coined by Gattefosse, and was introduced to Britain in the late 1950s by Marguerite Maury, who was a student of Gattefosse. She developed Gattefosse's work to a more practical conclusion, by combining the use of essential oils with massage. She developed specialised massage techniques and the 'individual prescription', a more holistic approach in which essences are chosen according to the physical and emotional needs of the client. Marguerite Maury devoted the rest of her working life to teaching and training therapists in the special techniques she had developed. Her first lectures in Britain were to beauty therapists, who began to introduce essential oils with massage to help relieve stress and skin conditions.

Today, thanks to Marguerite Maury, aromatherapy has developed from being used mainly in perfumes and cosmetics to a more holistic treatment – true aromatherapy lies in selecting and blending oils individually for each client. But, despite its ancient origins, aromatherapy is still in its infancy in the UK. Research into this fascinating therapy is still taking place, as it becomes recognised as a complementary therapy, and is used in many hospitals and clinics across the country.

Since the original publication of this book in 1997, the aromatherapy market has progressed commercially (it is worth at least £24 million in the UK alone) but has also developed to become available on the National Health Service (NHS).

Around 40 per cent of GP practices offer their patients access to some form of non-conventional treatment, such as aromatherapy.

The aromatherapy industry is currently working towards regulation of the profession.

The Aromatherapy Organisations Council (AOC) was instrumental in setting up the Aromatherapy Regulation Working Group, which is moving towards voluntary self-regulation for aromatherapy and therefore provides the basis for eventual statutory regulation.

Aromatherapists in the UK currently work at different levels, from the provision of aromatherapy massage for stress relief and relaxation, through to the clinical approach of aromatherapy employed in a health care setting.

A range of National Occupational Standards is being defined to encompass the broad spectrum of practitioners who work in different settings, and are subject to an approval process through the Standards Setting Body Skills for Health and the Aromatherapy Organisations Council.

Details of the progress of regulation of the aromatherapy profession may be accessed by visiting www.aromatherapy-regulation.org.uk.

Aromatherapy and the NHS

The Department of Health issued guidelines in June 2000 on Complementary and Alternative Medicine (CAM) to Primary Care Groups, listing the benefits of aromatherapy as 'promoting relaxation, treating painful muscular conditions and reducing anxiety ... with some evidence to support its beneficial use in intensive care, cardiac and palliative care'.

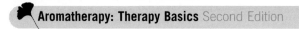

The advice given to primary care practitioners wishing to refer their patients to a complementary therapist recommends that they seek a therapist with an AOC recognised qualification.

Aromatherapy and stress management

Occupational health departments in some hospitals and private organisations offer a range of services to their staff including stress management, aromatherapy and massage.

Projects such as these have proved extremely popular with staff in helping them to manage stress levels and improve staff morale.

Aromatherapy and cancer care

NHS cancer patients can now choose to receive a wide range of treatments, including aromatherapy, from complementary therapy teams in around 90 per cent of hospitals and hospices throughout the country.

The Bristol Cancer Help Centre

The Bristol Cancer Help Centre was founded in 1980 with the aim to pioneer a holistic approach to cancer care.

The centre runs educational courses and workshops that are aimed at health professionals, complementary therapists and lay people.

Aromatherapists who wish to extend their professional knowledge and develop to work with clients with cancer may undertake a series of professional courses run at the Centre. Details are available by visiting their website at www.bristolcancerhelp.org.

BACUP is an organisation dedicated to helping people live with cancer. They provide a wide range of support services and publish a list of informative publications including 'Complementary Therapies and Cancer'.

For details visit www.cancerbacup.org.uk. Their address is BACUP, 3 Bath Place, Rivington Street, London EC2A 3JR.

Aromatherapy in its Diversity of Care

Aromatherapy is such a wide-reaching subject that there are endless examples of client groups it may benefit.

Aromatherapy is used to help many members of the community including children with common childhood problems such as eczema, people with depression, elderly clients with dementia, couples with infertility problems, clients with anxiety, patients with high blood pressure, to name but a few.

For reference to articles on specific subjects and examples of how aromatherapy has helped, visit www.internethealthlibrary.com.

Research and Funding

Despite there being a greater acceptance of complementary medicine among health care professionals, there is still a lack of funding in the UK for research into non-orthodox methods of health care, such as aromatherapy.

NHS primary care groups and health authorities are reluctant to spend large sums of money on non-conventional approaches, without research-based evidence of effectiveness and efficacy.

This indicates a growing need for a national strategy for complementary medicine research, where funding may be allocated to give credibility to clinical trials in subjects such as aromatherapy on a sufficient number of patients.

Serious funding is needed to support the many processes involved in research protocols (providing network resources, training researchers, disseminating information, and monitoring the development of research through to implementation). See Chapter 12.

Aromatherapy today represents a de-stressing programme for the whole person and its extensive uses may complement orthodox treatments to help restore the body's balance. May this wonderful therapy continue to soothe our stressed lives and progress well into the 21st century.

Self-assessment Questions

1. Define the term 'aromatherapy'.

----

2. Why is aromatherapy often referred to as a 'holistic therapy'?

----

3. Give a brief outline of how aromatherapy developed from its more primitive use in Egyptian times to become a complementary therapy today.

CHAPTER 2

Safety in Aromatherapy

> *Essential oils have been used in the form of the whole plant for thousands of years for medicinal and cosmetic purposes, but when distilled from the plant they become a hundred times more concentrated. Their physical, physiological and pharmacological effects on the body are therefore increased, and knowledge of safe levels of usage are of paramount importance to a practising aromatherapist.* **Proportion** *is the key to a safe aromatherapy practice.*

✱ A competent aromatherapist needs to understand and apply all safety precautions to the use of essential oils, to ensure a safe and effective treatment.

Objectives

By the end of this chapter you will be able to relate the following knowledge to your work as an aromatherapist:

✱ contra-indications to aromatherapy

✱ hazards associated with essential oils

✱ safety precautions and guidelines when practising aromatherapy

✱ storage and safe handling of essential oils.

As the benefits of aromatherapy are generally so far reaching, it is tempting to assume that it will be effective for everyone. However, there are certain medical conditions that may contra-indicate treatment or cases that may require special care and handling.

Contra-indications may be classified in the following way:

✱ general contra-indications that affect all treatments

✱ those that are localised and which affect specific areas

✱ those that require special care.

Key Note

For insurance purposes and in order to work within strict ethical guidelines, an aromatherapist must ensure that if a client is currently undergoing medical treatment or is under hospital care, then advice is sought from the client's GP before any form of treatment is undertaken.

If you are in any doubt about the suitability of your client for aromatherapy treatments, always seek advice from the client's GP before commencing treatment.

Contra-indications and Cautions for Aromatherapy Massage

It should be remembered that clients with medical conditions might present with factors that may increase the effects of the essential oils used. However, it should also be stressed that there are a multitude of essential oils whose effects may also benefit a client's condition, for instance Lavender essential oil combined with the relaxing effects of an aromatherapy massage may help to lower a client's blood pressure and improve their general circulation.

Medical advice should always be sought for a client with a medical condition to reduce the risk of adverse effects, and guidelines for choice of essential oil should be based on common sense and reliable clinical data, if available.

It should also be considered that, whilst massage may be contra-indicated for certain conditions, other forms of treatment might be suitable (such as inhalation, compresses, skin creams and lotions etc).

Conditions that are contra-indicated to aromatherapy massage include:

Fever   in the case of a fever there is a risk of spreading infection due to the increased circulation created by a massage. During fever, body temperature rises as a result of infection.

Infectious diseases   (colds, flu, measles, tuberculosis, scarlet fever) these are contra-indicated due to the fact they are contagious.

Skin diseases   care should be taken to avoid the risk of cross infection and of spreading the infection.

Recent haemorrhage   haemorrhaging is excessive bleeding, which may be either internal or external. Massage should be avoided due to the risk of increasing blood spillage from blood vessels. If in any doubt, medical advice should be sought.

Conditions that may be contra-indicated or may require GP referral and an adaptation of treatment include:

Severe circulatory disorders and heart conditions   medical clearance should be sought as there is a risk that the increased circulation from the aromatherapy massage may overburden the heart and increase the risk of a thrombus or embolus. If medical clearance is given, the aromatherapy massage should be applied lightly and gently.

Essential oils such as Lavender and Marjoram may help a client with a heart condition as they are considered to be heart sedatives.

Thrombosis   medical clearance should be sought as there is a risk that the increased circulation from the aromatherapy massage may move a clot to the heart. If medical clearance is given, the massage should be applied lightly and gently.

High blood pressure   clients with high blood pressure should have a medical referral prior to aromatherapy massage even if they are on prescribed medication, due to their susceptibility to form clots.

Clients taking anti-hypertensive medication may be prone to postural hypotension and may feel light-headed and dizzy after treatment. Care should therefore be taken to assist a client off the couch and ensure that they get up slowly.

Once medical clearance is obtained, aromatherapy massage should be generally soothing and relaxing.

Several essential oils are said to help lower blood pressure and these include Clary Sage, Lavender, Lemon, Marjoram and Sweet Orange.

Low blood pressure   care should be taken with a client suffering from low blood pressure when sitting or standing after massage due to the fact they may experience dizziness and could fall.

Care should be taken to avoid essential oils that are more sedative and help to lower blood pressure, in particular Lavender and Marjoram.

Epilepsy   medical advice should always be sought prior to massaging a client with a history of epilepsy. *If clearance is given, care should be taken to avoid the use of oils that are too stimulating on the nervous system or too deeply relaxing to reduce the risk of convulsions.*

An important consideration is the choice of aroma as some types of epilepsy may be triggered by smells.

Diabetes   clients with diabetes require medical referral as they may also be prone to arteriosclerosis, high blood pressure and oedema. Pressure should be carefully monitored due to any loss in sensory nerve function resulting in the client being unable to give accurate feedback regarding pressure.

If the client is receiving injections, care should be taken to avoid aromatherapy massage on recent injection sites. Clients should also have their necessary medications with them when they attend for treatment, in the event of an emergency.

Cancer   medical advice and guidance should always be sought before carrying out an aromatherapy treatment on a client who has a cancerous condition. There is a theoretical risk that certain types of cancer may spread through the lymphatic system and that aromatherapy massage may aid in the metasis of the cancer.

Common sense tells us that lymph flow will not be stimulated any more by gentle massage than it will by the muscular contraction caused by normal body movement. There is therefore no reason to believe that gentle massage will cause cancer cells to spread, which would not otherwise have done so.

Advice should always be sought from the consultant/medical team in charge of the client's care before proceeding to massage a client with cancer.

Aromatherapy massage treatment, if advised by the medical team, and requested by the client, should be light and short and will usually be offered to specific areas such as the hands, face and feet.

When massaging a cancer patient, care should be taken to avoid areas of the body receiving radiation therapy, close to tumour sites or lymph glands and areas of skin cancer.

It is well known that the use of certain essential oils and gentle aromatherapy massage can be beneficial to cancer patients in helping in palliative health care and in helping them to cope psychologically with their condition and alleviate some of the side effects of the cancer treatment.

Conditions that may present as a localised contra-indication and restrict treatment include:

Skin disorders some conditions may be exacerbated by aromatherapy massage. Some skin conditions, if inflamed, may need to be treated as a localised contra-indication.

Stress-related skin conditions in particular respond favourably to aromatherapy.

Recent scar tissue aromatherapy massage should only be applied to scar tissue once it has fully healed and can withstand pressure.

The use of cell regenerating essential oils such as Lavender, Frankincense and Neroli can help in healing and cell regeneration.

Severe bruising localised massage is contra-indicated in order to avoid discomfort and pain.

Varicose veins care should be taken to avoid direct pressure with massage on or around a varicose vein. If severe, medical clearance may be necessary as the client may be prone to thrombosis.

Gentle aromatherapy massage given proximally to the areas may help to reduce oedema and prevent venous and lymphatic stasis.

Cuts and abrasions these should be avoided as aromatherapy massage could further damage the healing tissue and expose the client and therapist to infection.

Recent fractures and sprains it is important to seek medical clearance before massaging a sprain or injury, due to the risk of increased vascular bleeding.

Undiagnosed lumps, bumps and swellings clients should be referred to their GP for a diagnosis. Aromatherapy massage may increase the susceptibility to damage in the area by virtue of pressure and motion.

Special factors to be taken into consideration before an aromatherapy massage and which may require special care include:

Asthma in general the use of specific essential oils with aromatherapy massage may help breathing difficulties such as asthma. Care would need to be taken to avoid allergies to essential oils or carrier oils and care may be needed in the positioning of the client.

Allergies and skin intolerances a patch test would need to be carried out before treatment commences in order to eliminate the risk of adverse reaction to the essential oils proposed for use.

Medication   the use of certain essential oils may exacerbate the excretion of drugs by speeding up the detoxification of the liver. However, a significant interaction between an essential oil and drugs is unlikely unless essential oils have been given in oral doses.

The interaction between essential oils and drugs is an area that remains unexplored and is largely undocumented, due to there being no yellow card system for recording reactions, as in traditional medicine.

Homeopathic preparations   there is no conclusive answer as to whether aromatherapy interferes with homeopathic treatment. Some believe the actions and strong odours of certain essential oils (such as Peppermint) may antidote homeopathic treatment, others feel that aromatherapy may enhance its actions.

If a client is undergoing homeopathic treatment at the time of an aromatherapy massage then it is sensible for the client to consult their homeopath to ensure that the proposed treatment you intend to offer is in synergy with the homeopathic preparations.

Abdominal treatment for women during menstruation   the abdominal area may be omitted from the aromatherapy massage during menstruation to avoid discomfort. However, some clients may find massaging the lower back helpful in offering pain relief and comfort.

Pregnancy   as essential oils will cross the placental barrier they have the potential to affect the foetus. Safe guidelines for treating pregnant women include:

* avoid treating any women with a poor obstetric history (bleeding, miscarriages) without advice from the client's GP/obstetrician
* avoid any form of treatment during the first trimester of the pregnancy
* use lower dilutions of essential oils (usually 1 per cent or less)
* avoid all oils considered to be emmenagogues and research known safety data to avoid potentially toxic essential oils that may be harmful to mother and foetus.

Migraine   some strong or heavy odours may precipitate or exacerbate the effects of a migraine. Careful choice of oils is needed in consultation with the client.

Children and babies   require special care and handling. A lower dilution of oils (1 per cent or less) should be used and care should be taken to avoid all toxic oils (recommended oils for children include Roman Chamomile, Lavender, Rose and gentle citrus oils such as Mandarin).

Key Note

Essential oils that are considered to be safe to use during pregnancy in a lower dilution (i.e. 1 per cent) include:

Bergamot, Chamomile (Roman and German)*, Cypress, Frankincense*, Geranium, Grapefruit, Lavender*, Lemon, Mandarin, Neroli, Orange, Patchouli, Petitgrain, Rose otto*, Sandalwood and Ylang Ylang.

* Avoid during first few months of pregnancy

The majority of essential oils when used correctly in aromatherapy treatments represent a negligible risk. However, it should be remembered that essential oils are very powerful and concentrated substances, and should therefore be employed with a great deal of care as inappropriate use may cause undesired effects.

There are three main types of hazard associated with essential oils:

* toxicity

* irritation

* sensitisation.

Toxicity

Toxicity is a broad term, which is used in aromatherapy to describe the hazardous effects associated with the misuse of essential oils. Toxic reactions depend on the amount of essential oils being used, the method of administration and the physiological status of the client being treated.

There are two main categories of toxicity:

* acute

* chronic.

Acute toxicity

This refers to the result of a short-term administration of a substance, and usually involves a single high lethal dose. Acute toxicity may be sub-categorised into the following classifications:

* *Acute oral toxicity* – this literally means 'poisoning' when an essential oil is taken orally in a high lethal dose; this may result in death. So far, all serious reported cases of poisoning have arisen after oral ingestion of essential oils. Aromatherapy massage is therefore unlikely to give rise to such a serious risk as poisoning.

* *Acute dermal toxicity* – high levels of essential oils are applied and readily absorbed through the skin to cause systemic toxicity, which could cause damage to the liver and kidneys (these are the two major organs of the body to filter out unwanted toxic substances from the bloodstream).

Chronic toxicity

This is the repeated use of a substance over a period of weeks, months or years, and is used to describe the adverse effects produced in the skin or elsewhere in the body, either by external or internal use.

Adverse effects of chronic toxicity may include headaches, nausea, minor skin eruptions, and lethargy.

> ## Key Note
>
> The degree of toxicity in aromatherapy depends not only on the amount of essential oil used but also on its route of administration. Oral administration represents by far the highest risk of toxicity and therefore should NOT be used in aromatherapy unless under the direction of a qualified Medical Practitioner.
>
> It should be noted that external use of essential oils is the only established form of treatment in the UK at this present time. The amount of essential oil absorbed from oral administration in a 24-hour period is 8–10 times greater than in massage. It can therefore be concluded that any acute toxicological effects are likely to be less pronounced following dermal application than by oral administration.

As toxicity is dose-dependent, the only risk of toxicity with essential oils is concerned with overuse and overdose.

Dose-dependency also refers to the size of the individual being treated: special care is required when treating a baby or young child as they are much more likely to develop toxicity with a much smaller amount of essential oil than an adult.

Most toxic effects of essential oils are attributable to known chemical compounds. It is therefore essential for aromatherapists always to refer to known safety data of essential oils before using them.

A useful reference is *Essential Oil Safety: A Guide for Health Professionals* by Robert Tisserand and Tony Balacs (ISBN 0-443-05260-3).

Common examples of toxic essential oils include:

* Aniseed
* Arnica
* Mugwort
* Pennyroyal
* Sassafras
* Savory
* Thuja
* Wintergreen
* Wormwood.

Phototoxicity

This term refers to a photochemical reaction that takes place in the skin by the combination of a phototoxic oil and ultra-violet rays. It may result in a mild colour change, to rapid tanning and hyperpigmentation. Depending on the severity of the photochemical reaction, it may cause blistering or deep weeping burns.

The most common phototoxic agents in essential oils are *furocoumarins* (such as bergaptene in bergamot oil), which, upon exposure to sunlight (natural or artificial), can cause adverse skin reactions.

Common examples of essential oils that may present a risk of phototoxicity include:

* Bergamot (expressed – a method of production for citrus oils in which oil is expressed from the rind of the fruit)

* Lemon (expressed)

* Bitter Orange (expressed)

* Lime (expressed)

* Grapefruit (expressed).

The risk of phototoxicity can be eliminated or at least reduced to safe levels by adhering to the following safe practice:

* Use furocoumarin free bergamot (FCF) (see Key Note below) or distilled citrus oils that are non-phototoxic.

* Use sunscreen to reduce the potential effect of phototoxicity.

* Ensure that the area treated is covered and is not exposed to strong sunlight (natural or artificial) for at least eight hours following treatment with phototoxic oils.

Key Note

Bergamot is an example of a fractionated essential oil (i.e. one that has part of the chemical composition removed). Research has shown that bergamot containing less than one part per 1,000 of bergaptene (the substance known to cause phototoxicity) is safe to use on the skin. Bergamot FCF indicates that the phototoxic bergaptene has been removed or reduced to a safe level to use on the skin.

Irritation

This is the most common type of reaction of the skin to essential oils, and is caused when a substance such as an essential oil reacts with the mast cells of the skin and releases histamine.

The term *irritation* refers to localised inflammation that may affect the skin and mucous membranes, and results in itchiness as well as varying degrees of inflammation.

Irritation is dose-dependent, and so reaction is directly proportional to the amount used in treatment.

> ## Key Note
>
> The risk of irritation is most acute when essential oils are used undiluted or are used in high concentration. It is interesting to note that there appears to be a wide tolerance variation between individuals. Reactions are idiosyncratic (they only affect a small majority of people).
>
> As the mucous membranes are thinner and much more fragile than the skin, they are in danger of becoming irritated. Care must be taken with the amount of essential oils used for inhalations (due to the risk of irritating the respiratory tract). Essential oils should never be used via the rectum, vagina or mouth, due to the potential high risk of irritation to the mucous membrane of the urino-genital and alimentary tract organs. Essential oils should be kept well away from the eyes.

Common examples of essential oils representing a risk of irritation include:

* Cinnamon Leaf
* Clove Bud
* Clove Stem
* Clove Leaf
* Red Thyme
* Wild Thyme.

Note: Some more common essential oils may occasionally cause irritation if used undiluted on the skin.

Carcinogenic substances

Little is known about the risk of dermally applied potentially carcinogenic substances found in essential oils, such as safrole and estragole.

Some essential oils that contain small components of estragole and safrole are considered safe for use in aromatherapy at the maximum external concentration (use 1–2 per cent) but which should not be taken in oral dosages include: Fennel, Basil (low estragole), Ho Leaf (camphor/safrole CT), Nutmeg (i.e. Indian), Cinnamon Leaf and Star Anise.

Essential oils that Tisserand and Balacs advise should be avoided altogether in aromatherapy due to the carcinogenic potential include Ravensara anisata, Sassafras, Basil (high estragole), Tarragon (French), Camphor (brown), Calamus (Indian), Tarragon (Russian) and Camphor (yellow).

Sensitisation

This is an allergic reaction to an essential oil, and usually takes the form of a rash, similar to the reaction of the skin to urticaria. For sensitisation to occur, the allergen (i.e. an essential oil) must penetrate the skin and will involve an immune response by the release of histamine. It will cause an inflammatory reaction, brought about by the cells of the immune system (T-lymphocytes) becoming sensitised. Upon first exposure to the substance, the effects on the skin will be slight if at all; but on repeated application of the same substance, the immune system will produce a reaction similar to dermal inflammation and the skin may appear blotchy and irritated.

Sensitisation is not dose-dependent, and so it is not dependent on concentration. Intolerance may build up on repeated contact with a sensitising oil, or after one application.

Common examples of essential oils that may cause sensitisation include:

* Cinnamon (bark, leaf and stem)
* Ginger
* Lemon
* Lemongrass
* Lime
* Melissa
* Bitter Orange
* Peppermint
* Teatree
* Thyme.

Degradation of essential oils can lead to increased hazards. For instance, the oxidation of the chemical compound terpenes makes the essential oils more likely to cause skin sensitisation.

Patch testing

Patch testing is an effective way of predicting allergic reaction to essential oils.

Key Note

When dealing with clients with sensitive skin or skin with intolerances, it is wise to perform a patch test for both irritation and sensitisation of a potentially hazardous oil.

In order to test for irritation, apply a couple of drops of the essential oil to the inside of a plaster, place on the inside of the forearm and leave unwashed for 24 hours. Repeat the test a second time if you wish to test for sensitisation.

Prior to working on areas such as the face and neck where cosmetics have been used, it is advisable to ensure that all preparations have been removed before applying essential oils, due to the risk of cross-sensitisation occurring on areas that are building up sensitivity to cosmetics. A positive result (which may indicate irritation) may result in erythema, itching and swelling. For female clients, skin sensitivity generally increases just before a menstrual period and at ovulation, due to hormonal influences at this time.

Safety Precautions When Using Essential Oils

When using essential oils, the following safety precautions should be followed to ensure a safe, effective treatment with no adverse effects to either the client or to the therapist:

* Always work in a well-ventilated area.

* Keep and dispense essential oils away from the treatment area, preferably in a separate room.

* In between clients, air the treatment room and allow yourself a break of at least five minutes.

* Keep essential oils away from the eyes and other sensitive parts of the face.

* Always undertake a detailed consultation to ascertain a client's physical and psychological condition, along with any medication they may be taking.

* If your client presents a medical condition, always refer them to their GP before treating.

* Never take essential oils by mouth, rectum or vagina, unless under medical instructions.

* Never apply undiluted oils to the skin.

* Always use in sensible proportions.

* Avoid prolonged use of the same essential oil.

* If your client suffers with sensitive skin or allergies, it is advisable to carry out a simple skin test before using an essential oil for the first time.

* Always label all blends.

* Always keep a full and accurate record of the essential oils used on a client and their dilution.

* Never use an essential oil with which you are not familiar.

Safe Handling and Storage

Due to the fact that essential oils are concentrated substances and are toxic if misused, great care must be taken when storing and handling them:

* Store in dark glass bottles in normal to cool temperatures (approx. 65 °F/18 °C), with lids secured tightly to prevent evaporation.

* Store all essential oils out of the reach of children.

* Keep essential oils away from naked flames, as they are highly flammable.

* Take care when handling essential oil bottles to ensure that your skin does not come into contact with the undiluted oil, and so that you avoid transferring it from your hands to more sensitive parts (e.g. nose, face and neck).

* Wash hands thoroughly in between clients, to remove as much of the oil as possible.

* Avoid using oils if your skin is cracked and sore.

All essential oils sold for professional and home use should carry safety precautions in their labelling.

An independent body, the Aromatherapy Trade Council (ATC), was formed in 1992 by responsible essential oils suppliers.

The ATC:

* represents the aromatherapy essential oil industry in the UK.

* works proactively and effectively to ensure the sector is represented on all relevant statutory and non-statutory bodies, thereby influencing policy decisions at all levels of regulation and legislation.

* co-ordinates the views of the industry and represents them to the appropriate authority.

* obtains policy statements on, and interpretation and clarification of, the current regulatory position from the relevant competent authorities.

* establishes guidelines for safety, labelling and packaging for the aromatherapy trade.

* acts as a focal point for public and media enquiries on the sector.

* supplies sound information and advice to members and the public.

* promotes genuine high standards of quality in essential oils within the industry by education and public relations.

* has a policy for the random testing of its members' oils.

* publishes a General Information Booklet and a list of current members.

* gives guidelines as to what is permissible on the labels and in promotional material for aromatherapy products and publishes a leaflet entitled 'Responsible Marketing & The Medicines Control Agency'.

* offers a service to its members and potential suppliers of aromatherapy products to review labels and publicity material prior to printing to ensure they comply with the complexities of the law.

* liaises with the media on a regular basis to ensure good public relations, with offers either to write aromatherapy articles or to check journalists' articles for accuracy, so that sound information is provided to the public for their protection.

* works closely with the aromatherapy profession through the Aromatherapy Organisations Council (AOC) and other organisations:

   – to promote training and education;

   – to advise on regulatory issues relating to the aromatherapy trade;

   – to promote the responsible use of aromatherapy products;

   – to ensure the needs of the profession are appropriately served by the aromatherapy trade.

The Code of Practice recommended by the ATC includes the following:

The ATC has a policy for the non-ingestion of essential oils and for the general public only to use essential oils externally unless advised otherwise by a qualified aromatherapist. It is for this reason that all members are required to state clearly on the labels of their products 'For external use only' or 'Do not take internally'.

Responsible marketing – warnings and information

All promotional material should give clear guidelines as to how essential oils are to be used, giving recommended dilutions where necessary. To comply with the consumer safety requirement, the following warnings and information must be printed on the consumer product label:

* Clear instructions for use, e.g. add 5 drops of essential oil to 10 ml of carrier or 6 drops in a bath.

* Keep away from children and eyes.

* Do not take internally or apply undiluted to the skin.

* The quantity supplied, e.g. 10 ml.

* The company name.

* Company address or post code.

* Batch code number.

* Botanical and common name of the plant.

Regulation of essential oils and aromatherapy products

In order to comply with consumer legislation, essential oil suppliers have a duty to carry out responsible marketing.

The Medicines Act 1968 states that no medicinal claims can be made on labels, promotional material or advertised regarding products that have not been licensed.

Essential oils are well regulated by legislation; and the diverse end products of the aromatherapy industry (cosmetics and pre-blended oils) fall under different regulatory regimes.

From the safety control viewpoint, they fall into three potential categories:

1 Herbal remedies (that is, medicinal products) exempt from licensing when mixed, administered or sold by aromatherapists in the course of their business. No medicinal claims may be made since essential oils are not licensed products. The Medicines Act Leaflet (MAL.8) gives guidance on their regulation and can be accessed through the Medicines Control Agency's (MCA) website at **www.open.gov.uk/mca/ourwork/licensingmeds/herbalmeds/herbalmeds.htm**

2 Cosmetics, e.g. ready-blended aromatherapy products using essential oils/carrier oils, bath oils, etc., sold to the public, are subject to the Cosmetic Product (Safety) Regulations 1996. A guide to these regulations is available free of charge from your local Trading Standards Office.

3 General Products, i.e. essential oils sold to the public, are subject to the General Product Safety Regulations 1994, a copy of which is also available from Trading Standards.

There are therefore legal controls to protect the consumer:

* The MCA deals with manufacturers who make medicinal claims without an appropriate marketing authorisation (medicines' licence).

* Trading Standards deal with those who sell adulterated essential oils or incorrectly label their products.

Key Note

There is often confusion between the terms 'essential oil' and 'aromatherapy oil'.

Essential oils are extracted by distillation or, in the case of citrus oils, by expression from a single botanical species. Once the primary process of distillation or expression has been completed, nothing further should be added.

An aromatherapy oil is a blend of undefined percentages consisting of diluents (usually vegetable oils) and essential oils (and sometimes with absolutes) and is suitable for use without further dilution.

Key Note

In order to comply with consumer legislation, essential oils suppliers have a duty to carry out responsible marketing.

The Medicines Act 1968 clearly states that no medicinal claims can be made on labels, promotional material or advertisements regarding products that have not been licensed. This means that no aromatherapy product can make remedial claims if it relates to a specific disease or adverse condition.

Task

Complete the following table to identify the type of hazard associated with essential oils.

Hazard	Description
	Essential oil taken orally in a high lethal dose; can be fatal.
	High levels of essential oils are applied to skin, and cause systemic toxicity; affects liver and kidneys.
	Photochemical reaction that takes place in skin by combination of phototoxic oil and ultra-violet rays.
	Localised inflammation of skin, caused by essential oil reacting with the mast cells of skin, releasing histamine. Affects skin and mucous membrane and is dose-dependent.
	Allergic reaction to an essential oil, involves an immune response by releasing histamine and causes the T-lymphocytes to become sensitised. Reaction may be slight on first exposure to allergen but on repeated exposure skin may appear blotchy and irritated. Is not dose-dependent.

✳ Table 2: Hazards associated with essential oils ✳

Self-assessment Questions

1. Why is safety an important factor when using essential oils?

----

2. State ten safety precautions to be taken into account when practising aromatherapy.

----

3. State five conditions that may contra-indicate aromatherapy treatment, stating the action required in each case.

----

4. *State five safety factors to be taken into account when storing essential oils.*

---

5. *State five essential oils that are unsafe to use in aromatherapy.*

---

6. *List five safety factors that should be on the label of essential oil bottles sold for professional and home use.*

CHAPTER 3

The Extraction of an Essential Oil

The most important ingredient in aromatherapy is the essential oil, a highly concentrated volatile substance obtained from various parts of the aromatic plant. Despite being used extensively in the food industry as flavourings and in the cosmetic industry in perfumes, when used in aromatherapy they have the ability to penetrate the skin and be absorbed into the bloodstream. Utmost care must therefore be taken in their application to the body.

✳ A competent aromatherapist must know the nature and effects of essential oils in order to understand the physical and psychological effects of aromatherapy treatments.

Objectives

By the end of this chapter you will be able to relate the following knowledge to your work as an aromatherapist:

✳ the nature and origins of essential oils

✳ methods of extracting essential oils

✳ factors to consider when storing essential oils

✳ common forms of adulteration

✳ factors to consider when purchasing essential oils

✳ vocabulary associated with an essential oil.

Essential oils play an important role in the plant, as they are responsible for their fragrance and are the most concentrated part of its vital force or energy. A typical essential oil consists of over 100 organic chemical compounds, which influence its aroma, therapeutic effects and in certain cases its potential hazards (such as irritation, sensitisation or toxicity).

Essential oils are present in the plant in special cells, and may be extracted from various parts of the plant matter; for example, the leaves, flowers, fruit, grass, roots, wood, bark, gums and blossom.

Essential oils are usually present in minute quantities in comparison to the mass of the whole plant, and may exist in the plant material in concentrations ranging from 0.01 to 10 per cent.

The nature of essential oils is therefore complex as they exhibit the following various characteristics:

* *Highly concentrated*   when extracted from the raw material, an essential oil can become 100 times more concentrated.
* *Highly aromatic*   the individual aroma of the essential oil becomes more defined after being extracted from the plant.
* *Highly volatile*   they evaporate quickly on contact with the air.
* *Liquid*   most are liquid, although some are solid at room temperature (e.g. rose).
* *Mainly colourless or pale yellow*   although some are more obviously coloured (e.g. blue chamomile).
* *Insoluble in water*   they will only dissolve in alcohols, fats, oils and waxes.

Key Note

Owing to their sensitivity, it is advisable to store essential oils in a dark, airtight glass container in cold conditions, in order to maintain their optimum therapeutic activity. It is also important to ensure that the 'head space' above the oil is not too great, to avoid oxidation and degradation.

If buying essential oils in larger quantities than 15 ml, it is advisable to decant the oil into several smaller dark glass bottles to reduce the headspace above the oil's surface to help prevent oxidation.

Storage Factors Associated with Essential Oils

* **Dark bottles** are used to reduce the amount of light access to essential oils.
* **Airtight bottles** are used to reduce the access of air to the oils, to prevent further oxidative reactions taking place and to prevent the escape of more volatile components.
* **Glass containers** are used because they do not react chemically (unlike plastic, which may either leach out of the plastic into the oils, or out of the oils into the plastic container).
* **Cool conditions** are necessary to reduce the enzymatically controlled chemical reactions that take place with the 'living' essential oils. The rate of reactions is doubled for over 10 °C rise in temperature. Therefore essential oils are kept in cool conditions, as their shelf life is greatly enhanced.

Key Note

It is helpful if droppers supplied in essential oil bottles are of different sizes according to the viscosity of the oil concerned. Good internal droppers will have a groove on one side. With the groove uppermost the oil will come out of the bottle with a slow drip; with the groove downwards the oil will come out as a fast drip.

Methods of Extraction

As essential oils are extracts from plants, they are subject to several processes and can vary according to:

* where they are grown
* the climate
* the altitude
* the soil
* the agricultural methods
* the time of harvesting.

It is therefore very important that the starting material used to produce the essential oil represents the natural biochemistry of the plant, in order that an oil with the highest grade of quality may be produced.

Due to their differences in distribution there are several methods of producing essential oils:

* steam distillation
* solvent extraction
* expression
* enfleurage
* super-critical carbon dioxide extraction
* phytonic process.

Steam distillation

This is the oldest and most established method of extracting the essential oil from the plant. Plant material, such as flowers, and leaves needs very little preparation prior to being distilled, except that they need to be cut up to allow the cell walls of the plant to rupture and the volatile oil to escape.

* The process involves placing the prepared plant material, such as leaves and flowers, into a large stainless steel container called a *still*.
* Steam is then passed under pressure through the plant material, and the heat causes the globules of essential oil to burst open, and the oil quickly evaporates.
* The steam and the essential oil vapour then pass out from the top of the still and along a glass tube, which is water-cooled, in order to condense the water back into a liquid.
* It is then a relatively simple process to separate the essential oil from the water, since the two do not mix. The water distillate left after extraction of the essential oil is a valuable by-product, and is used as a flower water or hydrolat.

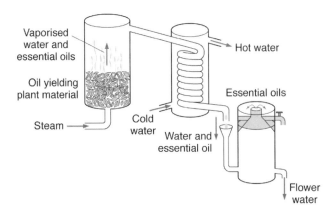

✳ Figure 1: Steam distillation of essential oils ✳

Key Note

During the distillation process, only the very small molecules can evaporate, and it is *these* tiny molecules that constitute the essential oil.

The heat and water used in the distillation process are potentially harmful to the fragile chemical constituents of the essential oil, and can alter the quality of the original plant material. Using low pressure steam and heat, pure water and fresh materials during the distillation process can therefore ensure the production of the best quality and 'environmentally friendly' essential oil.

Variations of steam distillation

Variations of steam distillation use low heat and take a long period to distil a batch of oil. These methods can result in a better quality oil as the larger molecules can be drawn out of the plant material.

High temperature methods, favoured for modern mass production, can produce essential oils more efficiently, lowering the cost, but some of the bouquet can be lost with this method.

Solvent extraction

This process involves placing the plant material in a vessel and covering it with a volatile solvent such as petroleum ether, benzene or hexane, which is used to extract the odoriferous part of the material.

✳ The mixture is slowly heated and the solution is filtered off, resulting in a dark coloured paste called a *concrete* (this is a combination of wax and essential oil) or it may be a resin, which is a solid or semi-solid natural product, which may be prepared or natural (e.g. exudation from a tree).

✻ The concrete then undergoes a second process, when it is agitated with alcohol and chilled in order to recover most of the aromatic liquid and remove the plant waxes.

✻ The alcohol is then evaporated leaving a high quality flower oil or absolute, which is fragrance/perfume material obtained from this process.

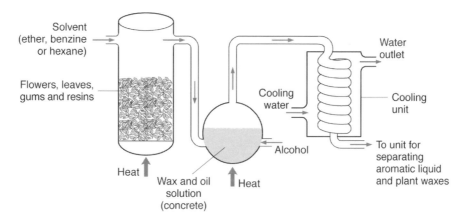

✻ Figure 2: Solvent extraction✻

Key Note

Solvent extraction is used extensively in the perfumery industry and produces some of the finest flower fragrances. There is an element of controversy regarding the suitability of the use of absolutes in aromatherapy, as they contain solvent residues, which may cause adverse skin reactions.

Expression

This process is used solely for the citrus family and therefore may be used for what may more accurately be called *essences*.

✻ The oil from the citrus fruit lies in little sacs under the surface of the rind and simply needs to be pressed out.

✻ The process of expression used to be carried out by hand, where the rind was literally squeezed by hand until the oil glands in the rind burst. This was then collected in a sponge and squeezed into a container once the sponge was saturated.

✻ Expression is now carried out by machinery in a process known as *scarification*, and is usually produced in a factory that produces fruit juice in order to maximise the profit from the whole fruit.

> ## Key Note
> As no heat is used in the process of expression, the aroma and the delicate chemical structure of the essence extracted is almost identical to that contained within the rind of the fruit.

Enfleurage

This is the traditional method used to extract the finest quality essences from delicate flowers such as rose and jasmine, which continue to generate oil after harvesting. It is a very long labour-intensive process, and hence is virtually obsolete now.

* The process involves using wooden glass rectangular frames and spreading a thin layer of purified fat onto the glass.
* Freshly picked petals are then sprinkled over the fat and the glass sheet frames are stacked in tiers. The essence from the flower is then absorbed into the fat.
* The faded petals are removed after 24 hours, after which fresh petals are laid over the fat.
* The process is repeated until the fat is saturated with enough essence from the flower – at this stage it is known as a *pommade*.
* The pommade is then diluted in alcohol to obtain the extracts, and the alcohol evaporates, leaving only the oil. The remaining fat is used commercially to make soap.

Fewer than 10 per cent of essential oils are produced by this method and enfleurage has been largely replaced by solvent extraction.

Super-critical carbon dioxide extraction

This is a relatively new method of extracting essential oils and uses compressed carbon dioxide at very high pressure to extract the essential oil from the plant material.

The essential oils produced by this method are reputed to be of exceptional quality and to be more like the essential oil from the plant in terms of their quality and stability. The disadvantage with using this method is that the equipment used is not only massive, but also extremely expensive to use.

The phytonic process

This is a newly developed method of extracting essential oils from the plant, which uses environmentally friendly solvents that have the ability to capture the aromatic oils of the plants at or below room temperature. This ensures that the highly fragile and heat sensitive constituents of the essential oil are neither lost nor altered due to their extraction process. The oils produced by this method are known as 'phytol' oils.

Adulteration of Essential Oils

Unfortunately, due to the widespread popularity of essential oils, there is an increased practice of adulteration.

An adulterant is an impurity accidentally or deliberately introduced into a product, rendering it of inferior quality.

If an aromatherapist buys and uses sub-standard or adulterated products, they run the risk of not only minimising the efficacy of their treatment, but also of provoking potentially negative reactions from their clients.

Adulterations may take one of several forms:

* A very small quantity of the essential oils may be diluted in a spirit base and therefore is 'let down'.

* A quantity of the main chemical constituent may be added to the essential oil to 'stretch' it; for example, linalool is commonly added to Clary Sage, Lavender, Neroli and Rosewood.

* Synthetic aromatic substances may be added, resulting in a fabricated oil.

* An essential oil from a cheaper plant may be added, for example, Lemon to Bergamot or Citronella to Melissa.

* Some of the chemical constituents may be removed; these oils are known as *fractionated* oils. For example, a main chemical constituent of essential oils such as terpenes can be removed, which is useful for the perfume industry.

Key Note

Essential oils have a highly complex chemistry, which makes it impossible to reproduce them synthetically. Synthetic substances or reconstructed oils are in general very successful for perfumery and may also have specific uses in flavourings and pharmaceuticals, but in aromatherapy, essential oils are designed for vibrational healing and therefore it cannot be stressed highly enough that only the *purest* oils in their natural state will give the desired therapeutic effects. Remember that the greater the interference with the chemical constituents of the essential oil, the fewer therapeutic effects it will have. Adulterated oils can have undesired effects such as causing skin irritation and sensitisation.

Factors to Consider When Purchasing Essential Oils

It is imperative to buy essential oils from a reputable supplier. Factors to consider when making your choice include:

Quality

The plant itself, its harvest method, the type of soil used and the country of origin will all play a part in the final determination of quality. If you are in doubt about the quality of an oil, it is advisable to ask suppliers for information concerning the origins of the oil and methods used to test for purity.

Key Note

A supplier or importer of essential oils may use a method of testing for purity called Gas Liquid Chromatography, which is an accurate method of determining an oil's composition, and will reflect the chemical profile of the essential oil. It is often referred to as 'chemical fingerprinting' and is carried out on behalf of some essential oil companies in laboratories by specialist chemists.

Gas Liquid Chromatography will also highlight any undesirable substances, for example, trace contaminants in the plant such as biocides, herbicides or pesticides that have been used in its production.

Each essential oil tested is given a certification of conformity and a batch number to confirm its purity, if it meets the stringent laboratory tests.

Purity

A pure essential oil can be defined as one that has been produced from a botanical source and has not been modified in any way that alters its unique qualities.

Key Note

Reputable professional suppliers will take steps to ensure that the essential oils they produce are grown by organic means (i.e. without the use of chemical fertilisers and poisonous sprays). Organic producers meeting the required standards of production are awarded certificates by the Soil Association in Britain.

The production of organic essential oils

The principles of organic agriculture involve the minimal use of non-renewable resources, minimisation of pollution and damage to the environment, respect for animal welfare, minimal processing and minimal use of additives and processing aids.

In the UK, farmers must join a recognised organic association and the UK Soil Association is the most well known. Organic farming and food processing are regulated by EU law, which requires that any food labelled as organic must have been produced and processed according to the standards laid down in the EU Organic Regulation No 2092/92. This is implemented in the UK by the United Kingdom Register of Organic Food Standards (UKROFS), which controls and monitors the organic certification bodies. The organic certification bodies then inspect and certify organic producers, processors, importers and retailers.

Organic essential oil crops

In the UK, farmers must comply with all of the above regulations, even though essential oil crops are non-food.

During evolution plants had to defend themselves from predators and pests and one method was to incorporate in-built chemical warfare in the leaves, flowers, seeds, roots etc. Today we call these chemicals 'essential oils' and, in reality, they are the pesticide. This means that, when grown as crops, they may not need fungicides or insecticides.

Generally speaking, temperate climate essential oil plants are considered to be wild plants and this means that they have not been bred and selected for cultivation. As a result, they are not responsive to nitrogenous fertiliser and require very few crop inputs. Also, farmers do not use pesticides if there are no pests!

Organic farmers should not use any pesticides on essential oil crops. If a pesticide is needed it must be permitted (by the Organic Certification authority) and the name of the product and date of application recorded. These details should be available to the purchaser.

Organic farming also covers other aspects of agricultural knowledge and expertise. For example, for essential oil crops, the grower should select named botanical species for cultivation. Crop residues should be appropriately recycled and organic oils kept separate from any produced non-organically.

It has been difficult to detect pesticide residues in essential oils. However, data is now available that shows levels of organochlorine pesticides in various essential oils.

A checklist for buyers of organic essential oils

In reality, according to UKROFS, essential oils (called herbal oils by the EU) do not come under the EU Regulation 2092/92. This means that anyone can legally call any essential oil 'organic'. The purchaser should look for *organic certification*.

1. The grower (farmer) of the essential oil crop must be certified as organic by a recognised authority in the country of production.

2. The method of organic agriculture in that country must be equivalent to the legislation described by the EU Regulation 2092/92. In other words, the conversion period and permitted crop inputs should be the same.

3. If the grower (farmer) undertakes the essential oil extraction, the processing method must also be certified as organic.

4. If a third party undertakes the crop processing, their methods should be certified as organic.

5. Soil Association Certification traces the name of the grower in the country of origin, the botanical name of the crop species/variety, the date of harvest, the date of processing, the method of processing, and the method of storage. This information should be available to the purchaser (within the parameters of commercial confidentiality).

6. The Organic Certification procedure should detail any crop inputs. The point here is that although some pesticides are permitted for food crops, they should not be used at all for essential oil crops particularly if they are volatile.

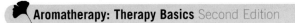

It is possible for an essential oil supplier to register their company with a recognised organic authority. This still means that all of the above information should be available. The Soil Association only recognises non-UK certification bodies if they meet the same (equivalent) standards. Some countries do produce genuine *certified organic* essential oils. Some do not and careful scrutiny is needed.

Some certified organic essential oils may be a little more expensive due to the increased costs to farmers of removing weeds from the crops (usually by hand). Certain weeds may act as toxic botanicals if extracted with the essential oil crop (e.g. stinking mayweed, mugwort) and special care and knowledge is needed. For those requiring essential oils for their medicinal properties, wild collections should certainly be avoided.

Further information

Soil Association, 86 Colston Street, Bristol BS1 5BB. Tel 0117 929 0661

Dr Jane Collins, Mill House Certified Organic Medicinal and Aromatic Plant Farm and Research Centre, Eager Lane, Lydiate, Merseyside L31 4HS. Tel/Fax 0151 526 0139. drcollins@madasafish.com

Price

In general, the price of an essential oil reflects the yield of oil in the plant along with its production costs. Rose petals produce very little oil, which makes the essential oil fairly expensive, whereas eucalyptus gives a high yield and is relatively cheap. Price is not, however, an indication of purity or quality.

Odour

This will depend on the origin of the oil, its method of production and other factors concerning the oil such as storage, transport method, temperature, purity, age, quality and degree of nasal perception.

Best before date

This is important as essential oils are affected by age, light, heat and oxidation. It is useful to know either the production date or its expiry date, to assess its life expectancy to an aromatherapist.

> ## Key Note
>
> As most essential oils are affected by age, it is recommended that they are used within two years of first opening to avoid degradation. Citrus oils have a relatively short life and under good storage conditions will remain unchanged for up to a year.
>
> Despite this, some essential oils such as patchouli actually improve with age, and can remain unchanged for many years.
>
> It is also worth considering that once, produced, essential oils have a rather convoluted journey before reaching you, therefore a best before date is very useful in practice.

Origin

The part of the plant used and the country of production may reflect differences in essential oils such as composition, quality or price. Good suppliers' price lists will indicate the part or parts of the plant used to produce the oil along with its country of origin. Remember that the origin of the plant determines its character and chemical composition.

Botanical name of plant

As there are many species or variations of plants, which all exhibit different characteristics, it is important to know the botanical or Latin names of the plant to ensure their authenticity and original character and composition.

Safety

Choose essential oils bottles with child resistant closures.

Key Note

The best advice is to purchase your essential oils from a reputable professional supplier who is prepared to give you as much information as possible regarding the nature of the oils and their origins.

Most professional suppliers list a batch number on the essential oil bottle, which is useful to note when you want a repeat order of the same oil.

Although purity is high on the list of priorities when purchasing essential oils, it should be noted that there are no tests, including Gas Liquid Chromatography, which guarantee purity. Whilst Gas Chromatography will highlight any chemical imbalances in the oil that could not be possible in the natural essential oil, it cannot assess its exact chemistry as the precise chemical constituents of essential oils are still largely unknown.

A useful checklist when considering choosing an essential oil supplier is:

1 Do they provide comprehensive literature of their oil including botanical names, sources, etc?

2 Does your contact with them reflect they are knowledgeable about the oils; are they happy to answer your questions?

3 How much information is included regarding quality testing? Is there independent analysis of their oils?

4 Are the essential oils clearly and correctly labelled, with the recommended safety guidelines?

5 How safety conscious are they?

6 How efficient is their service?

Current EC Regulations are moving towards greater definition and more detailed information regarding the nature of essential oils in order that the consumer may expect to get:

✳ an essential oil or aromatic from a named botanical source and from a given origin

✳ an oil that has been tested and analysed by experts who can determine its quality.

Task

Complete the following table to identify the following terms used in connection with essential oils.

Term	Description
	Aromatic material (viscous or semi-solid perfume material) extracted from plants using solvent extraction.
	Solid or semi-solid dark-coloured paste; a combination of wax and essential oil.
	Volatile and aromatic liquid obtained by distillation or expression.
	A by-product of steam distillation.
	Solid or semi-solid natural product, may be prepared or natural (e.g. exudations from trees).

✳ **Table 3: Terms used to describe essential oils** ✳

Self-assessment Questions

1. Define an essential oil.

----

2. State five characteristics of an essential oil.

----

3. Why should essential oils never be used in their undiluted form?

----

4. Give a brief outline of the following methods of extracting essential oils:

   i) steam distillation

----

ii) solvent extraction

---

5. State five important factors to consider when purchasing essential oils.

---

6. State three common forms of adulteration of essential oils.

CHAPTER 4

The Essential Oils

Essential oils have many chemical components that reflect the life force of the plant, and they possess a variety of functions in the plant from which they are derived. These varied functions found within the oil are elements that, in the plant form, help to fight disease, stimulate growth and reproduction. It is not therefore unreasonable or illogical to expect those same elements to have a variety of functions on the human body.

Orthodox drugs are often very specific and have a single active principle, which is either isolated from the plant or synthetically constructed in a laboratory. Essential oils, however, are more holistic, as they work on several levels.

✳ A competent aromatherapist needs to know the therapeutic effect attributed to essential oils, to understand their effects on the body.

Objectives

By the end of this chapter you will be able to relate the following knowledge to your work as an aromatherapist:

✳ the origin, method of production and therapeutic properties of 40 common essential oils.

As you begin to study the many therapeutic effects of essential oils, you will begin to realise that each oil may be used to treat a variety of conditions, and that most conditions will respond positively to a number of oils.

Essential oils are diverse – there is a large spread of actions with many oils and a degree of overlap in the choice of oil for a particular condition. This is because of the complex chemistry of an essential oil. The chemical constituents of an essential oil are often closely related in their molecular structure to those of human cells and tissues and hormones: therefore, as well as having a direct action upon specific bacteria and viruses, the oils also act by stimulating and reinforcing the body's own defence mechanism.

The Essential Oils

Basil (Sweet)

A very effective oil, well known for its cephalic property and for its effects on the digestive and respiratory systems.

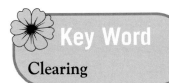

Key Word

Clearing

Botanical name:	Ocimum basilicum
Source:	flowering top and leaves of the herb
Method of production:	steam distillation
Aroma characteristics:	light, clear, sweet and slightly spicy
Odour intensity:	high
Note:	top
Blends well with:	Bergamot, Black Pepper, Clary Sage, Geranium, Lavender, Marjoram, Melissa, Neroli, Sandalwood

Energetic Profile
Towards the Yang (warm)

Therapeutic properties

* adrenal cortex stimulant
* analgesic
* antidepressant
* antiseptic
* antispasmodic
* carminative
* cephalic

* digestive
* emmenagogue
* expectorant
* febrifuge
* nervine
* stomachic
* tonic

Therapeutic uses

* **Circulatory system**   poor circulation

* **Digestive system**   dyspepsia, gastric spasms, hiccups, nausea

* **Endocrine system**   irregular periods, menstrual pain

* **Immune system**   coughs, colds, flu

* **Musculo-skeletal systems**   muscular aches and pains

* **Nervous system**   anxiety, depression, migraine, headaches, nervous tension

* **Respiratory system**   asthma, bronchitis

* **Skin care**   congested skins and acne

Psychological profile: Basil is useful for confusion, hysteria, lack of assertiveness, lack of self-worth, melancholia and vulnerability.

Summary

Safety data

* Avoid during pregnancy

* May cause sensitisation and irritation

* There have been recent concerns over the possible carcinogenic effects of methyl chavicol contained in the exotic Basil chemotype, therefore it is advisable to use the French Basil chemotype therapeutically

See Photo 1 on page 91.

Benzoin

Benzoin is a very useful oil for inflammatory skin conditions due to its soothing properties, and for any condition in which fluid needs to be expelled from the body.

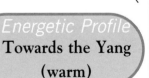

Key Word

Soothing

A very valuable oil for general stress relief and nervous tension.

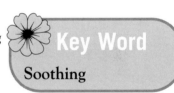

Botanical name:	Styrax benzoin
Source:	gum from the trunk of the tree
Method of production:	solvent extraction
Aroma characteristics:	sweet vanilla-like
Odour intensity:	high
Note:	base
Blends well with:	Bergamot, Cypress, Frankincense, Juniper, Lavender, Lemon, Myrrh, Orange, Petitgrain, Rose and Sandalwood

Energetic Profile
Towards the Yang (warm)

Therapeutic properties

* anti-inflammatory
* antiseptic
* astringent
* carminative

* diuretic
* sedative
* tonic (heart)
* vulnerary

Therapeutic uses

* **Circulatory system**   poor circulation
* **Digestive system**   indigestion, flatulence
* **Immune system**   coughs, sore throats
* **Musculo-skeletal system**   muscular aches and pains
* **Nervous system**   nervous exhaustion, nervous tension
* **Respiratory system**   asthma, bronchitis
* **Skin care**   cracked or chapped skin
* **Urinary**   cystitis

Psychological profile: Benzoin is useful for nervous anxiety, depression, emotional exhaustion, feelings of loss, grief, loneliness and worry.

Summary

Safety data

Although Benzoin is categorised as non-toxic and non-irritant, it may cause sensitisation in some individuals.

See Photo 2 on page 91.

Bergamot

Bergamot is a very uplifting oil to both mind and body and is an invaluable choice for depression and stress-related conditions.

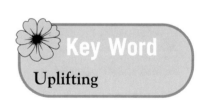

Key Word

Uplifting

Botanical name:	Citrus bergamia
Source:	peel of a small orange-like fruit
Method of production:	cold expression
Aroma characteristics:	light, delicate, spicy lemon/orange aroma with slight floral overtones, very refreshing and uplifting
Odour intensity:	medium
Note:	top
Blends well with:	the Chamomiles, Cypress, Eucalyptus, Geranium, Jasmine, Lavender, Lemon, Marjoram, Neroli, Palmarosa, Patchouli, Rose and Ylang Ylang

Energetic Profile
Towards the Yin (cool)

Therapeutic properties

* analgesic
* antidepressant
* antiseptic (pulmonary and genito-urinary)
* antispasmodic
* antiviral
* astringent
* carminative
* diuretic
* laxative
* parasiticidal
* rubefacient
* stomachic
* stimulant
* tonic
* vulnerary

Therapeutic uses

* **Digestive system**   dyspepsia, flatulence, colic, indigestion
* **Immune system**   colds
* **Nervous system**   anxiety, depression and stress-related problems
* **Respiratory system**   asthma, bronchitis, catarrh, coughs
* **Skin care**   acne, oily and congested skins
* **Urinary**   infections such as cystitis, thrush

Psychological profile: Bergamot is useful for anger, anxiety, depression, despair, grief, lack of confidence, lack of courage, nervous tension, negativity and worry.

Summary

Safety data

Due to the chemical constituents furocouramins (notably bergapten) Bergamot will increase photosensitivity of the skin. Care needs to be taken therefore to avoid contact with strong ultra-violet light or sunlight after using this oil. Alternatively, a bergapten-free (FCF) variety may be used.

See Photo 3 on page 91.

Black Pepper

Black Pepper is very stimulating to mind and body and is particularly effective on the muscular and digestive systems.

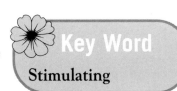

Key Word
Stimulating

Botanical name:	Piper nigrum
Source:	dried and crushed black peppercorns
Method of production:	steam distillation
Aroma characteristics:	spicy, hot and very sharp
Odour intensity:	high
Note:	middle
Blends well with:	Bergamot, Cypress, Frankincense, Geranium, Grapefruit, Lavender, Lemon, Palmarosa, Rosemary, Sandalwood, Ylang Ylang

Energetic Profile
Towards the Yang (warm)

Therapeutic properties

* analgesic
* antimicrobial
* antiseptic
* antispasmodic
* carminative
* detoxicant
* diuretic
* febrifuge
* laxative
* rubefacient
* stimulant
* stomachic
* tonic

Therapeutic uses

* **Circulatory system** poor circulation, anaemia
* **Digestive system** colic, constipation, diarrhoea, loss of appetite, nausea
* **Immune system** colds, flu, viral infections
* **Musculo-skeletal system** muscular aches and pains, poor muscle tone, joint pain and stiffness

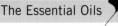

Psychological profile: Black Pepper is useful for indifference, lethargy, melancholy and mental fatigue.

Summary

Safety data

Black Pepper should be used in low concentration as it may cause skin irritation.

See Photo 4 on page 91.

Cajeput

Cajeput is a very effective expectorant and is helpful for respiratory problems. It is equally effective for circulation, muscles and joints in helping to ease muscular pains and stiffness.

Key Word

Releasing

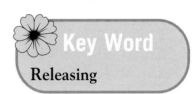

Botanical name:	Melaleuca leucadendron
Source:	leaves and twigs of tree
Method of production:	steam distillation
Aroma characteristics:	sweet and herbaceous: penetrating
Odour intensity:	high
Note:	top
Blends well with:	Bergamot, Geranium, Lavender, Rose, Rosewood, Thyme

Energetic Profile
Towards the Yang (warm)

Therapeutic properties

* analgesic
* antirheumatic
* antiseptic
* antispasmodic

* decongestant
* expectorant
* insectidical
* stimulant

Therapeutic uses

* **Digestive system**   colic, constipation, gastric spasms
* **Endocrine system**   menopausal problems, period pains
* **Immune system**   colds, flu
* **Nervous system**   neuralgia, headaches, toothache
* **Respiratory system**   pharyngitis, laryngitis and bronchitis
* **Musculo-skeletal system**   muscular aches and pains, joint pain and stiffness

Psychological profile: Cajeput is useful for helping to clear 'mental fog' and is effective when feeling mentally sluggish. It is also helpful for apathy, cynicism and those with a tendency to procrastination.

Summary

Safety Data

A powerful oil that has been reported to cause skin irritation, therefore it should be used in small proportions with care.

See Photo 5 on page 92.

Chamomile (Roman)

Best known for its soothing and calming effects on the emotions, as well as on many physical conditions, particularly those associated with the skin, digestive and nervous systems.

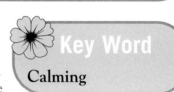

Key Word

Calming

Botanical name:	Anthemis nobilis
Source:	flower heads of herb
Method of extraction:	steam distillation
Aroma characteristics:	a strong apple-like aroma, sweet and warm
Odour intensity:	high
Note:	middle
Blends well with:	Bergamot, Clary Sage, Geranium, Jasmine, Lavender, Neroli, Rose

Energetic Profile
Towards the Yin (cool)

Therapeutic properties

* analgesic
* antidepressant
* anti-inflammatory
* antiseptic
* bactericidal
* carminative
* emmenagogue
* hepatic

* hypnotic
* nervine
* sedative (nerve)
* stimulates leucocytosis (production of white blood cells)
* stomachic
* tonic
* vulnerary

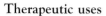

Therapeutic uses

* **Digestive system**   colic, dyspepsia, indigestion, nausea
* **Endocrine system**   menstrual and menopausal problems
* **Musculo-skeletal system**   muscular aches and dull pain
* **Nervous system**   depression, headache, migraine, insomnia, nervous tension and stress-related problems
* **Skin care**   allergies, dry and sensitive skins, inflammatory skin conditions
* **Urinary system**   cystitis

Psychological profile: Roman Chamomile is useful for anger, anxiety, fear, hysteria, irritability, melancholy, overactive mind, sensitivity, nervous tension, weepiness and excessive worry.

Summary

Safety data

It is advisable to avoid using Roman Chamomile in the early stages of pregnancy. Use in low concentrations as it may cause dermal irritation/sensitisation.

See Photo 6 on page 92.

Chamomile (German/Blue)

Blue Chamomile is a very effective oil in skin care, particularly on allergies and inflammatory skin conditions.

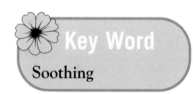

Key Word

Soothing

Botanical name:	Matricaria chamomilia
Source:	flower heads of herb
Method of production:	distillation
Aroma characteristics:	strong, sweetish, warm and herbaceous
Odour intensity:	very high
Note:	middle
Blends well with:	Benzoin, Bergamot, Clary Sage, Geranium, Jasmine, Lavender, Marjoram, Melissa, Patchouli, Rose, Ylang Ylang

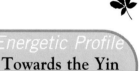

Energetic Profile
Towards the Yin (cool)

Therapeutic properties

* analgesic
* anti-inflammatory
* antispasmodic
* bactericidal
* carminative
* digestive
* emmenagogue

* febrifuge
* hepatic
* sedative (nerve)
* stimulates leucocytosis (production of white blood cells)
* stomachic
* vulnerary

Therapeutic uses: See Roman Chamomile

Psychological profile: See Roman Chamomile

Summary

Safety data

* See Roman Chamomile
* Use in small proportions to avoid adverse skin reactions.

Chamomile (Moroccan)

Moroccan Chamomile differs in its chemical and olfactory makeup from Roman and Blue Chamomiles and therefore does not share their extensive properties. It is generally quite soothing and calming on the nerves.

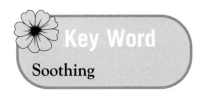

Key Word

Soothing

Botanical name:	Ormenis multicaulis
Source:	flowering tops of plant
Method of production:	steam distillation
Aroma characteristics:	sweet herbaceous aroma with a rich balsamic undertone
Odour intensity:	medium
Note:	middle
Blends well with:	Bergamot, Cypress, Lavender, Mandarin, Marjoram, Rosemary, Tangerine

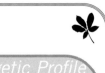

Energetic Profile
Towards the yin (cool)

Therapeutic properties

* antispasmodic
* emmenagogue

* hepatic
* sedative

Therapeutic uses

* **Digestive system** colic, colitis, liver and spleen congestion
* **Endocrine system** menstrual and menopausal problems
* **Nervous system** headache, migraine, insomnia
* **Skin care** sensitive skins, inflammatory skin conditions

Psychological profile: Moroccan Chamomile is helpful for frustration, irritability and nervous tension.

Summary

Safety data

Generally considered as non-toxic and non-irritant.

Clary Sage

Clary Sage is a deep muscle relaxant, which is helpful in aiding mind and body to relax simultaneously.

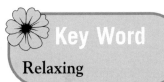

Key Word

Relaxing

Botanical name:	Salvia sclarea
Source:	flowering tops and leaves of the herb
Method of production:	steam distillation
Aroma characteristics:	heavy, leafy, nutty
Odour intensity:	medium
Note:	top to middle
Blends well with:	Bergamot, Cypress, Frankincense, Geranium, Grapefruit, Juniper, Lavender Sandalwood

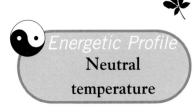

Energetic Profile

Neutral temperature

Therapeutic properties

* antidepressant
* antispasmodic
* carminative
* digestive
* emmenagogue
* euphoric
* hypotensive

* nervine
* parturient
* relaxant (muscle)
* stomachic
* tonic
* uterine

Therapeutic uses

* **Circulatory system** high blood pressure
* **Digestive system** colic, dyspepsia, constipation, flatulence, intestinal cramps
* **Endocrine system** pre-menstrual syndrome, menstrual problems (scanty or painful), menopause
* **Musculo-skeletal system** muscular aches and pains
* **Nervous system** migraine, insomnia, debility, stress-related problems
* **Respiratory system** asthma, bronchitis, throat infections
* **Skin care** acne and oily skins

Psychological profile: Clary Sage is useful for anxiety, depression (post-natal, pre-menstrual and menopausal), fear, guilt, moodiness, negativity, obsessional behaviour, panic, paranoia, rage, restlessness and worry.

Summary

Safety data

Avoid use of Clary Sage during pregnancy, and avoid combining use with alcohol consumption as it may cause drowsiness.

See Photo 7 on page 92.

Cypress

The key property of Cypress is that it is a powerful astringent, excellent for circulation and an effective 'hormonal' oil. Reputedly good for coughs and respiratory complaints (in France cough pastilles were once made from crushed Cypress cones).

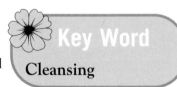

Key Word

Cleansing

Botanical name:	Cupressus sempervirens
Source:	needles, twigs and cones of the tree
Method of production:	steam distillation
Aroma characteristics:	pleasant smoky, forest aroma; clear and refreshing
Odour intensity:	medium
Note:	middle to base
Blends well with:	Benzoin, Bergamot, Clary Sage, Juniper, Lavender, Lemon, Orange, Pine, Rosemary, Sandalwood

Energetic Profile
Towards the Yin (cool)

Therapeutic properties

* antirheumatic
* antiseptic
* antispasmodic
* astringent
* deodorant
* diuretic

* febrifuge
* haemostatic
* hepatic
* sedative
* tonic
* vasoconstrictor

Therapeutic uses

* **Circulatory system**   poor circulation, varicose veins
* **Endocrine system**   menstrual problems, menopausal symptoms
* **Immune system**   coughs, flu
* **Musculo-skeletal system**   muscular aches and pains, joint pain
* **Nervous system**   nervous tension, irritability
* **Respiratory system**   asthma, bronchitis, whooping cough
* **Skin care**   acne, oily skin (and hair), excessive perspiration
* **Urinary system**   cystitis

Psychological profile: Cypress is useful for bereavement, confusion, despondency, emotional instability, frustration, impatience, irritability, lack of trust, mood swings, nervous tension, feelings of regret, self-loathing, sorrow and withdrawal.

Summary

Safety data

No specific precautions; generally considered to be non-toxic, non-irritant and non-sensitising.

See Photo 8 on page 92.

49

Eucalyptus

Eucalyptus is a very powerful oil, having powerful effects on the respiratory systems, and is an excellent agent in healing flesh wounds and external ulcers.

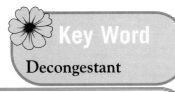

Key Word

Decongestant

Botanical name:	Eucalyptus globulus
Source:	leaves and twigs of the tree
Method of extraction:	steam distillation
Aroma characteristics:	clear, sharp, menthol, piercing and penetrating aroma; camphoraceous with a woody undertone
Odour intensity:	high
Note:	top
Blends well with:	Benzoin, Bergamot, Juniper, Lavender, Lemon, Lemongrass, Melissa, Pine, Rosemary, Thyme

Energetic Profile

Towards the Yang (warm)

Therapeutic properties

* analgesic
* antirheumatic
* antiseptic
* antiviral
* bactericidal
* decongestant
* depurative

* diuretic
* expectorant
* febrifuge
* rubefacient
* stimulant
* vulnerary

Therapeutic uses

* **Circulatory system**   poor circulation
* **Immune system**   coughs, flu
* **Musculo-skeletal system**   aches and pains, joint pain
* **Nervous system**   debility, headaches
* **Respiratory system**   asthma, bronchitis, catarrh, coughs, congestion in the head, sinusitis, sore throat
* **Skin care**   healing to the skin
* **Urinary system**   cystitis

Psychological profile: Eucalyptus is helpful for addiction, bitterness, guilt, loneliness, moodiness and resentment.

Summary

Safety data

Eucalyptus is a powerful oil and should be used in low concentrations. May antidote homeopathic preparations due to its strong odour.

See Photo 9 on page 93.

Fennel

Fennel is well known for its tonic action on digestion and for its detoxifying character.

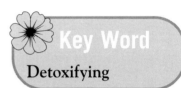

Key Word

Detoxifying

Botanical name:	Foeniculum vulgare
Source:	crushed seeds of the herb
Method of production:	steam distillation
Aroma characteristics:	aniseed; both floral and herby; slightly spicy
Odour intensity:	high
Note:	middle
Blends well with:	Geranium, Lavender, Lemon, Orange, Rose, Rosemary, Sandalwood

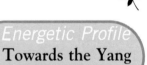

Energetic Profile

Towards the Yang (warm)

Therapeutic properties

* antiseptic
* antispasmodic
* carminative
* depurative
* detoxicant
* diuretic
* emmenagogue
* expectorant
* laxative
* stimulant
* stomachic
* tonic

Therapeutic uses

* **Circulatory system**   poor circulation, cellulite
* **Digestive system**   colic, constipation, dyspepsia, flatulence and nausea
* **Endocrine system**   pre-menstrual tension, menopausal problems, menstrual problems
* **Immune system**   coughs, flu
* **Musculo-skeletal system**   aches and pains, joint pain

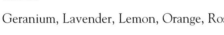

* **Nervous system**   nervous debility, headache
* **Respiratory system**   asthma, bronchitis, whooping cough
* **Skin care**   dull, oily and mature skins, tightens and tones the skin
* **Urinary system**   urinary tract infections

Psychological profile: Fennel is useful for boredom, emotional instability, emotional blockages, fear of failure, hostility, inability to adjust, lack of confidence, mental weakness, when feeling overburdened.

Summary

Safety data

* Use in moderation as Fennel is a powerful oil.
* Best avoided during pregnancy.
* Best avoided by epilepsy sufferers.
* It is recommended that sweet fennel is used in aromatherapy and NOT the bitter fennel, as it is more gentle.

See Photo 10 on page 93.

Frankincense

The chief uses of Frankincense are in skin care and respiratory infections.

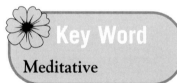

Key Word

Meditative

Botanical name:	Boswellia carteri
Plant origin:	resin of the tree
Method of extraction:	steam distillation
Aroma characteristics:	woody and spicy fragrance, with a rich balsamic undertone
Odour intensity:	high
Note:	middle to base
Blends well with:	Black Pepper, Geranium, Grapefruit, Lavender, Orange, Melissa, Myrrh, Patchouli, Pine, Sandalwood

Energetic Profile

Towards the Yin (cool)

Therapeutic properties

* anti-inflammatory
* antiseptic
* astringent
* carminative
* cytophylactic

* digestive
* emmenagogue
* expectorant
* sedative
* uterine

Therapeutic uses

* **Digestive system**   dyspepsia

* **Endocrine system**   menstrual problems

* **Immune system**   colds (head)

* **Nervous system**   anxiety, nervous tension, stress-related problems

* **Respiratory system**   asthma, bronchitis, catarrh, coughs, laryngitis, shortness of breath

* **Skin care**   regenerating on mature skins, acne, abscesses, scars and blemishes

* **Urinary system**   cystitis

Psychological profile: Frankincense is helpful for anger, apprehension, fear, grief, hopelessness, insecurity, irritability, lack of faith, nervous tension, remorse (dwelling on the past), tearfulness, vulnerability and worry. It helps to release emotional blockages.

Summary

Safety data

Best avoided in the first trimester of pregnancy. Frankincense is generally considered as non-toxic, non-irritant and non-sensitising.

See Photo 11 on page 93.

Geranium

Geranium is a very balancing and regulating oil, which tends to balance extremes, whether on the physical or emotional level.

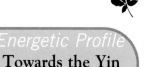

Key Word

Balancing

Botanical name:	Pelargonium graveolens	
Source:	flowers and leaves of the plant (pelargonium)	
Method of extraction:	steam distillation	
Aroma characteristics:	strong sweet and heavy aroma, reminiscent of Rose but with minty overtones	
Odour intensity:	high	
Note:	middle	
Blends well with:	Bergamot, Clary Sage, Grapefruit, Jasmine, Lavender, Neroli, Orange, Petitgrain, Rose, Rosemary, Sandalwood	

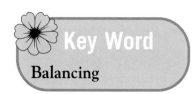

Energetic Profile
Towards the Yin (cool)

Therapeutic properties

* adrenal cortex stimulant
* antidepressant
* antihaemorrhagic
* anti-inflammatory
* antiseptic
* astringent

* cytophylactic
* diuretic
* haemostatic
* tonic (liver and kidneys)
* vulnerary

Therapeutic uses

* **Circulatory system** poor circulation, oedema
* **Endocrine system** pre-menstrual syndrome, menopausal problems
* **Lymphatic system** fluid retention, cellulite
* **Nervous system** nervous tension and stress-related problems
* **Skin care** effective on balancing all skin types, especially dry and oily. Effective for eczema, dermatitis, bruises and wounds

Psychological profile (balancing to the mind): Geranium is helpful for anxiety, confusion, depression (particularly linked to hormones), mental lethargy, moodiness, sadness and tearfulness.

Summary

Safety data

May cause irritation to sensitive skins, may cause restlessness if used excessively.

See Photo 12 on page 93.

Ginger

Ginger is a very stimulating oil, which has very positive effects on the muscular, digestive and nervous systems.

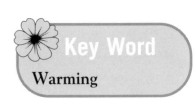

Key Word

Warming

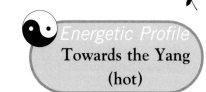

Botanical name:	Zingiber officinale
Source:	dried ground root of the plant
Method of production:	steam distillation
Aroma characteristics:	warm, woody and spicy
Odour intensity:	medium
Note:	middle
Blends well with:	Cajeput, Eucalyptus, Frankincense, Geranium, Lemon, Orange, Rosemary

Energetic Profile
Towards the Yang (hot)

Therapeutic properties

* analgesic
* antiseptic
* antispasmodic
* aperitif
* bactericidal
* carminative
* expectorant
* febrifuge
* laxative
* rubefacient
* stimulant
* stomachic
* tonic

Therapeutic uses

* **Circulatory system**   poor circulation, chilblains
* **Digestive system**   diarrhoea, indigestion, colic, flatulence, loss of appetite, nausea
* **Immune system**   colds (runny), catarrh, flu
* **Musculo-skeletal system**   aches and pains, muscular fatigue, joint pain
* **Nervous system**   nervous exhaustion
* **Respiratory system**   coughs, sore throat

Psychological profile: Ginger is helpful for apathy, burnout, confusion, lack of direction, lack of focus, loneliness, resignation and sadness.

Summary

Safety data

May cause irritation to sensitive skin; use in low concentrations.

See Photo 13 on page 94.

Grapefruit

Grapefruit is a very effective oil for stimulating the lymphatic system. It is very uplifting and will help depression and general stress-related conditions.

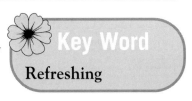

Key Word

Refreshing

Botanical name:	Citrus paradisi
Source:	fresh peel of the fruit
Method of production:	cold expression
Aroma characteristics:	fresh, sweet, sharp and refreshing
Odour intensity:	medium
Note:	top
Blends well with:	Bergamot, the Chamomiles, Frankincense, Geranium, Jasmine, Lavender, Palmarosa, Rose, Rosewood, Ylang Ylang

Energetic Profile

Towards the Yin (cool)

Therapeutic properties

* antiseptic
* astringent
* bactericidal
* depurative
* diuretic
* stimulant
* tonic

Therapeutic uses

* **Circulatory system** poor circulation
* **Digestive system** abdominal distension, constipation, nausea
* **Lymphatic system** fluid retention, cellulite
* **Immune system** coughs, colds, flu
* **Musculo-skeletal system** muscular fatigue, rheumatic pain
* **Nervous system** nervous exhaustion, headaches, depression
* **Skin care** acne, congested and oily skins
* **Urinary system** cystitis

Psychological profile: Grapefruit is helpful for depression, feelings of envy, fear, grief, lack of confidence and resentment.

Summary

Safety data

Skin irritation could occur if exposed to strong sunlight within 12–24 hours of treatment.

See Photo 14 on page 94.

Jasmine

Jasmine is most notably used for its effects on the reproductive system and the skin. Culpeper stated in his herbal, 'The oil is good for hard and contracted limbs, it opens, warms and softens the nerves and tendons'.

Key Word

Comforting

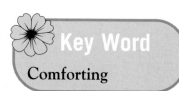

Botanical name:	Jasminum officinalis
Source:	fragrant white flowers of the shrub or vine
Method of extraction:	solvent extraction
Aroma characteristics:	very sweet, flowery and heavy aroma
Odour intensity:	very high
Note:	base
Blends well with:	Bergamot, Frankincense, Geranium, Orange, Mandarin, Melissa, Neroli, Palmarosa, Rose, Rosewood, Sandalwood, Tangerine

Energetic Profile

Neutral temperature

Therapeutic properties

* antidepressant
* anti-inflammatory
* antiseptic
* antispasmodic
* aphrodisiac

* expectorant
* parturient
* sedative
* uterine

Therapeutic uses

* **Endocrine system**   reproductive problems, menstrual pain, labour pain
* **Musculo-skeletal system**   muscular aches and pains, stiffness
* **Nervous system**   depression, nervous exhaustion, stress-related problems
* **Respiratory system**   coughs, colds, laryngitis
* **Skin care**   effective on all skin types, especially hot, dry and sensitive skins

Psychological profile: Jasmine is helpful for confusion, fear, depression, inhibition, lack of confidence, lack of self-worth, lack of interest, lack of trust, nervous tension and sadness.

Summary

Safety data

No known hazards if used in sensible proportions.

See Photo 15 on page 94.

Juniper

Juniper is a detoxifying oil that works effectively on an emotional and physical plane.

Key Word
Cleansing

Botanical name:	Juniperus communis
Source:	fresh ripe berries of the bush/evergreen tree
Method of extraction:	steam distillation
Aroma characteristics:	clear, refreshing, slightly woody aroma
Odour intensity:	medium
Note:	middle
Blends well with:	Benzoin, Bergamot, Cypress, Frankincense, Geranium, Grapefruit, Lavender, Lemongrass, Melissa, Orange, Rosemary, Sandalwood

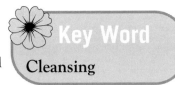

Energetic Profile
Towards the Yang (hot)

Therapeutic properties

* antirheumatic
* antiseptic
* antispasmodic
* astringent
* carminative
* depurative
* detoxicant

* emmenagogue
* nervine
* rubefacient
* stimulant
* stomachic
* tonic
* vulnerary

Therapeutic uses

* **Circulatory system**   poor circulation
* **Endocrine system**   menstrual problems
* **Lymphatic system**   fluid retention, tissue toxication
* **Muscular system**   muscular aches and pains, stiffness
* **Nervous system**   anxiety and nervous tension, stress-related problems
* **Skin care**   effective for acne, congested and oily skins

Psychological profile (cleansing to the mind and spirit): Juniper is useful for addiction, confusion, feeling of worthlessness, feeling of being emotionally drained, guilt, fear, obsession, restlessness and withdrawal.

Summary

Safety data

* Best avoided during pregnancy.
* Use in moderation as it can be very stimulating.

See Photo 16 on page 94.

Lavender

Lavender is a universally balancing oil and best known for its versatility, being equally effective on a wide range of conditions.

Key Word

Balancing

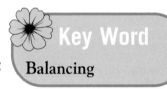

Energetic Profile
Towards the Yin (cool)

Botanical name:	Lavendula officinalis/augustifolia
Plant origin:	fresh flowering tops of the evergreen woody shrub
Method of extraction:	steam distillation
Aroma characteristics:	powerful herbal/floral aroma
Odour intensity:	medium
Note:	middle
Blends well with:	Bergamot, Chamomiles, Clary Sage, Geranium, Jasmine, Lemon, Lemongrass, Mandarin, Orange, Patchouli, Pine, Rosemary, Sandalwood, Thyme

Therapeutic properties

* analgesic
* antidepressant
* antirheumatic
* antiseptic
* antispasmodic
* antiviral
* bactericidal
* carminative

* cytophylactic
* decongestant
* diuretic
* emmenagogue
* hypotensive

* insecticidal
* nervine
* sedative
* vulnerary

Therapeutic uses

* **Circulatory system**   high blood pressure, heart conditions
* **Digestive system**   colic, dyspepsia, flatulence, nausea
* **Hormonal system**   pre-menstrual syndrome
* **Immune system**   colds, flu
* **Muscular system**   muscular aches and pains, joint pain
* **Nervous system**   depression, headache, insomnia, migraine, nervous tension and stress-related problems
* **Respiratory system**   asthma, bronchitis, coughs, sinusitis
* **Skin care**   all skin types, very healing and regenerating on all skins

Psychological profile: Lavender is helpful for anger, anxiety, despondency, depression, emotional instability, fear, hysteria, impatience, irritation, mood swings, negative thoughts, panic, paranoia and worry.

Summary

Safety data

Lavender is generally considered as non-toxic, non-irritant and non-sensitising and is best avoided during the early stages of pregnancy.

See Photo 17 on page 95.

Lemon

Lemon is a refreshing and cooling oil: its key function is in strengthening the immune system.

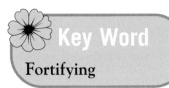
Key Word

Fortifying

Botanical name:	Citrus limonum
Source:	outer part of the fresh peel of the fruit
Method of extraction:	cold expression
Aroma characteristics:	refreshing sharp citrus aroma
Odour intensity:	medium to high
Note:	top
Blends well with:	Bergamot, the Chamomiles, Eucalyptus, Fennel, Frankincense, Ginger, Juniper, Neroli, Rose, Sandalwood, Ylang Ylang

Energetic Profile

Towards the Yin (cool)

Therapeutic properties

* antirheumatic
* antiseptic
* antispasmodic
* astringent
* carminative
* depurative
* diuretic
* febrifuge
* haemostatic
* hypotensive
* insecticide
* laxative
* rubefacient
* stimulates leucocytosis (production of white blood cells)
* stomachic
* tonic

Therapeutic uses

* **Circulation system**   poor circulation
* **Digestive system**   dyspepsia, bloatedness
* **Immune system**   colds, flu and infections
* **Respiratory system**   asthma, bronchitis, catarrh, sore throat
* **Skin care**   especially effective for oily skins

Psychological profile: Lemon is helpful for confusion, fear, mental fatigue and worry.

Summary
Safety data

May cause skin irritation and sensitisation in some individuals. The expressed essential oil is phototoxic; do not use on skin exposed to direct sunlight.

See Photo 18 on page 95.

61

Lemongrass

Lemongrass is a very powerful antiseptic, useful in combating infection. A valuable stress-relieving oil with a pleasant fresh aroma.

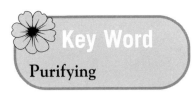

Key Word

Purifying

Botanical name:	Cymbopogon citratus
Source:	fresh and partially dried aromatic grass
Method of production:	steam distillation
Aroma characteristics:	sweet and lemony; fresh grassy aroma
Odour intensity:	medium to high
Note:	top
Blends well with:	Frankincense, Geranium, Jasmine, Lavender, Neroli, Palmarosa, Rosemary, Teatree

Energetic Profile

Towards the Yin (cool)

Therapeutic properties

* analgesic
* antidepressant
* antiseptic
* astringent
* bactericidal
* carminative
* deodorant
* digestive
* diuretic
* febrifuge
* nervine
* tonic

Therapeutic uses

* **Digestive system**   colitis, flatulence, indigestion
* **Immune system**   colds, flu and infections
* **Musculo-skeletal system**   tired aching muscles, fatigue
* **Nervous system**   nervous exhaustion, headaches, stress-related conditions
* **Respiratory system**   sore throat, fever
* **Skin care**   especially effective for oily skins, acne, open pores. Effective for excessive perspiration

Psychological profile: Lemongrass is helpful for lack of assertiveness, lack of mental clarity, lack of focus and judgement, nervous exhaustion and nervous tension.

Summary

Safety data

This oil is best used in low proportions, as it has the potential to cause dermal irritation/sensitisation.

See Photo 19 on page 95.

Mandarin

Mandarin is a very mild oil that is an excellent choice for pregnant women and children.

Key Word

Gentle

Botanical name:	Citrus nobilis
Source:	outer peel of the fruit
Method of production:	cold expression
Aroma characteristics:	delicate, sweet, tangy aroma with floral undertones
Odour intensity:	low to medium
Note:	top
Blends well with:	Basil, Bergamot, Black Pepper, the Chamomiles, Grapefruit, Lavender, Lemon, Marjoram, Neroli, Palmarosa, Petitgrain, Rose, Rosemary

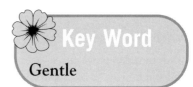

Energetic Profile
Towards the Yin (cool)

Therapeutic properties

* antispasmodic
* cytophylactic
* digestive
* sedative
* tonic

Therapeutic uses

* **Digestive system** flatulence, loss of appetite, colitis, constipation
* **Endocrine system** pregnancy, pre-menstrual tension
* **Nervous system** anxiety, depression, nervous tension, stress-related problems
* **Skin care** all skin types; particularly effective on stretch marks and scarring

Psychological profile: Mandarin is helpful for anxiety, dejection, dwelling on the past, feelings of emptiness, grief, nervous tension, over-excitability, restlessness and shyness.

Summary

Safety data

May be phototoxic, so it is best to avoid exposure to strong sunlight/ultra-violet light following treatment.

See Photo 20 on page 95.

Marjoram (Sweet)

Marjoram is a powerful muscle relaxant that allows the mind and body to relax simultaneously. It has a particularly soothing, warming and fortifying effect on disorders of the digestive, muscular, nervous and respiratory systems.

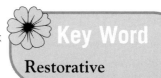

Key Word

Restorative

Botanical name:	Origanum marjorana
Plant origin:	dried leaves/flowering tops of herb
Method of extraction:	steam distillation
Aroma characteristics:	deeply penetrating, peppery, nutty, spicy and warming aroma
Odour intensity:	medium
Note:	middle
Blends well with:	Bergamot, the Chamomiles, Cypress, Lavender, Mandarin, Orange, Rosemary, Rosewood, Ylang Ylang

Energetic Profile
**Towards the Yang
(warm)**

Therapeutic properties

* analgesic
* antiseptic
* antispasmodic
* antiviral
* arterial vasodilator
* carminative
* digestive

* emmenagogue
* expectorant
* hypotensive
* laxative
* nervine
* rubefacient
* sedative (heart)

Therapeutic uses

* **Circulatory system**   high blood pressure, heart conditions
* **Digestive system**   colic, constipation, dyspepsia, flatulence
* **Hormonal system**   menstrual problems, pre-menstrual syndrome

* **Immune system**   colds
* **Muscular system**   muscular aches and stiffness, joint pain
* **Nervous system**   headaches, migraine, insomnia, nervous tension and stress-related problems
* **Respiratory system**   asthma, bronchitis, coughs

Psychological profile: Marjoram is helpful for anxiety, depression, fear, grief, loneliness and nervous tension.

Summary

Safety data

Best avoided during pregnancy.

See Photo 21 on page 96.

Melissa

Melissa is particularly associated with nervous disorders, the heart and the emotions, and for digestive and respiratory complaints of nervous origin.

Key Word

Comforting

Botanical name:	Melissa officinalis
Source:	leaves and flowering tops of the herb
Method of production:	steam distillation
Aroma characteristics:	sweet and lemon-like, with floral overtones
Odour intensity:	medium to high
Note:	middle
Blends well with:	The Chamomiles, Frankincense, Geranium, Ginger, Jasmine, Juniper, Lavender, Marjoram, Neroli, Rose, Rosemary, Ylang Ylang

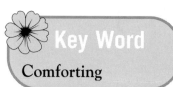
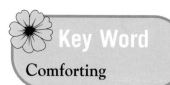

Energetic Profile
Towards the Yin (cool)

Therapeutic properties

* antiallergenic
* antidepressant
* antispasmodic
* carminative
* digestive
* febrifuge

* hypotensive
* nervine
* sedative
* stomachic
* tonic
* uterine

Therapeutic uses

* **Circulatory system** high blood pressure, palpitations

* **Digestive system** flatulence, gastric spasms, nausea, dyspepsia

* **Endocrine system** pre-menstrual tension, painful menstruation

* **Nervous system** migraines, headaches, anxiety

* **Respiratory system** asthma, colds, rapid breathing

* **Skin care** all skin types; particularly effective on very sensitive/allergic skin types.

Psychological profile: Melissa is helpful for grief, hypersensitivity, mental blocks, nervous tension, negativity, panic and shock.

Summary

Safety data

* Best avoided during pregnancy.

* May cause sensitisation and dermal irritation (avoid use with very sensitive skins).

* Best used in low dilutions only.

* Due to its cost Melissa is one of the most frequently adulterated oils commercially.

See Photo 22 on page 96.

Myrrh

Myrrh, like Frankincense, is an effective oil for respiratory and skin conditions.

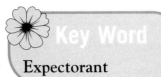

Key Word

Expectorant

Botanical name:	Commiphora myrrha
Source:	the gum from the trunk (oleoresin)
Method of production:	a) resinoid by solvent extraction and b) steam distillation from the crude myrrh
Aroma characteristics:	smoky and musky
Odour intensity:	high
Note:	base
Blends well with:	Benzoin, Frankincense, Lavender, Orange, Patchouli, Sandalwood

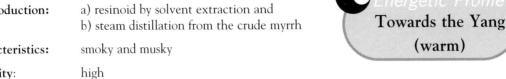

Energetic Profile

Towards the Yang (warm)

Therapeutic properties

* antiseptic
* astringent
* diuretic
* emmenagogue
* expectorant

* stimulant
* stomachic
* tonic
* uterine
* vulnerary

Therapeutic uses

* **Endocrine system**   pregnancy, pre-menstrual tension
* **Nervous system**   anxiety, depression, nervous tension, stress-related problems
* **Respiratory system**   coughs, bronchitis, sore throats
* **Skin Care**   all skin types; particularly effective on mature skins. Is very healing for cracked and chapped skin

Psychological profile: Myrrh is helpful for fear and uncertainty about the future, agitation, restlessness and where there is a tendency to overreact emotionally.

Summary

Safety data

Myrrh is best avoided during pregnancy.

See Photo 23 on page 96.

Neroli

Neroli is a wonderfully effective oil for stress relief and is one of the most effective oils for emotional shock.

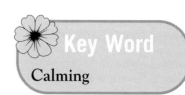

Key Word

Calming

Botanical name:	Citrus aurantium
Source:	freshly picked orange blossom flowers of the evergreen tree
Method of extraction:	steam distillation (a concrete and absolute are also produced by solvent extraction)
Aroma characteristics:	very sweet, floral aroma with a bitter undertone
Odour intensity:	medium
Note:	middle to base
Blends well with:	Benzoin, Bergamot, Geranium, Jasmine, Lavender, Lemon, Orange, Palmarosa, Petitgrain, Rose, Rosemary, Sandalwood, Ylang Ylang

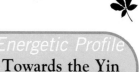

Energetic Profile
Towards the Yin (cool)

Therapeutic properties

* antidepressant
* antiseptic
* antispasmodic
* bactericidal
* carminative
* cytophylactic
* digestive
* nervine
* sedative
* tonic

Therapeutic uses

* **Circulatory system** poor circulation

* **Digestive system** colic, flatulence, stress-related digestive problems such as irritable bowel syndrome

* **Hormonal system** pre-menstrual syndrome

* **Nervous system** anxiety, depression, nervous tension

* **Skin care** effective for all skin types especially the dry, sensitive and mature skins

Psychological profile (reliever of extreme stress): Anxiety, apprehension, desperation, emotional trauma, fear and nervous tension.

Summary

Safety data

Neroli has no known hazards.

See Photo 28 on page 98.

Orange (Sweet)

Sweet Orange is a very 'smiley' oil, which can help to dispel nervous tension, whether purely emotional or linked to a physical ailment.

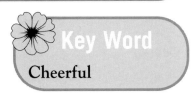

Key Word

Cheerful

Botanical name:	Citrus sinensis
Plant origin:	outer peel of fruit
Method of extraction:	cold expression
Aroma characteristics:	sweet fruity aroma, zesty and warm
Odour intensity:	medium
Note:	top to middle

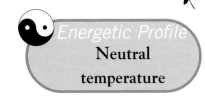

Energetic Profile

Neutral temperature

Therapeutic properties

* antidepressant
* antiseptic
* antispasmodic
* carminative
* digestive

* febrifuge
* sedative
* stomachic
* tonic

Therapeutic uses

* **Digestive system**   indigestion, constipation, stress-related disorders such as irritable bowel syndrome

* **Immune system**   colds and flu

* **Lymphatic system**   fluid retention

* **Nervous system**   nervous tension and stress-related problems

* **Skin care**   effective for dull, congested and oily skins

Psychological profile (comforting and warming to the spirit): Sweet Orange is helpful for anxiety, depression and emotional exhaustion.

Summary

Safety data

Sweet Orange has no known hazards.

See Photo 24 on page 97.

Palmarosa

Palmarosa is an excellent skin hydrator and regenerator and therefore is an effective choice in skin care.

Key Word

Regenerating

Botanical name:	Cymbopogon martinii
Source:	fresh, or dried grass, and leaves of the herbaceous plant
Method of production:	steam or water distillation
Aroma characteristics:	sweet, floral aroma; slightly dry with a hint of Rose
Odour intensity:	low to medium
Note:	top
Blends well with:	Bergamot, Geranium, Jasmine, Lavender, Melissa, Orange, Petitgrain, Rose, Rosewood, Sandalwood, Ylang Ylang

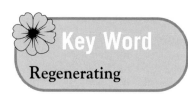

Energetic Profile

Towards the Yin (cool)

Therapeutic properties

*	antirheumatic	*	digestive
*	antiseptic	*	febrifuge
*	antiviral	*	hydrating
*	bactericidal	*	stimulant (digestive and circulatory)
*	cytophylactic	*	tonic

Therapeutic uses

* **Musculo-skeletal system** stiff muscles and joints
* **Nervous system** anxiety, depression
* **Skin care** all skin types; particularly effective on dry and mature skins

Psychological profile: Palmarosa is helpful for emotional trauma, feelings of being restricted or trapped or when feeling listless.

Summary

Safety data

Palmarosa has no known hazards.

See Photo 25 on page 97.

Patchouli

Patchouli is very useful in skin care, being a very effective cell regenerator. Unlike other oils, Patchouli seems to improve with age.

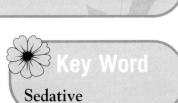

Key Word

Sedative

Botanical name:	Pogostemon cablin
Source:	dried leaves of the perennial bushy herb
Method of production:	steam distillation
Aroma characteristics:	earthy, sweet and spicy; strong, deep and exotic
Odour intensity:	high
Note:	base
Blending tip:	Due to the fact that Patchouli is highly odorous, it is advisable to use it sparingly in a blend.
Blends well with:	Bergamot, Black Pepper, Clary Sage, Frankincense, Geranium, Ginger, Lavender, Lemongrass, Myrrh, Neroli, Pine, Rose, Rosewood, Sandalwood

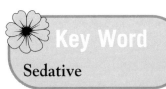

Energetic Profile

Neutral temperature

Therapeutic properties

* antidepressant
* antiseptic
* aphrodisiac
* astringent
* cytophylactic
* deodorant
* diuretic
* febrifuge
* insecticide
* sedative
* tonic

Therapeutic uses

* **Circulation system** poor circulation
* **Lymphatic system** fluid retention
* **Immune system** colds, flu and infections
* **Nervous system** depression, nervous exhaustion, stress-related conditions
* **Skin care** especially effective for oily skins, excessive perspiration, healing to cracked skin, skin infections

Psychological profile: Patchouli is helpful for anxiety, apprehension, depression, indecision, insecurity, mood swings and negativity.

Summary

Safety data

Patchouli is generally regarded as non-toxic, non-irritant and non-sensitising.

See Photo 26 on page 97.

Peppermint

Peppermint is a very stimulating oil to both mind and body and is therefore an excellent choice for mental and physical fatigue. It is also well known for its effects on the digestive and respiratory systems.

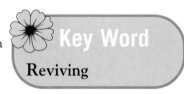

Key Word

Reviving

Botanical name:	Mentha piperita
Plant origin:	stems and leaves of the herb
Method of extraction:	steam distillation
Aroma characteristics:	strong, sharp piercing menthol aroma
Odour intensity:	medium to high
Note:	top
Blends well with:	Benzoin, Cypress, Lavender, Mandarin, Marjoram, Orange, Pine, Rosemary

Energetic Profile
**Towards the Yin
(cool)**

Therapeutic properties

* analgesic
* anti-inflammatory
* antiseptic
* antispasmodic
* antiviral
* cephalic
* decongestant

* emmenagogue
* expectorant
* febrifuge
* hepatic
* nervine
* stimulant
* vasoconstrictor

Therapeutic uses

* **Digestive system** colic, cramp, dyspepsia, flatulence and nausea
* **Immune system** colds and flu
* **Muscular system** muscular pain, joint pain
* **Nervous system** headaches, migraine, nervous stress
* **Respiratory system** asthma, bronchitis, sinusitis
* **Skin care** congested skins

Psychological Profile: Peppermint is helpful for depression and mental fatigue.

Summary
Safety data

Use in moderation as it is a very stimulating oil. May cause sensitisation due to menthol constituent. It is

* best avoided during pregnancy
* best avoided by those suffering with epilepsy or heart disease
* best avoided if homeopathic remedies are being taken.

See Photo 27 on page 97.

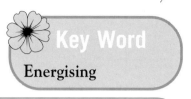

Petitgrain

Petitgrain is a very refreshing oil that has very beneficial effects on digestion and minor stress-related conditions.

Key Word

Energising

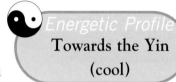

Energetic Profile
Towards the Yin (cool)

Botanical name:	Citrus aurantium
Source:	leaves and twigs of the tree
Method of production:	steam distillation
Aroma characteristics:	fresh, invigorating, slightly floral aroma with a woody herbaceous undertone (resembles Neroli but is slightly more bitter)
Odour intensity:	medium
Note:	middle to top
Blends well with:	Bergamot, Geranium, Lavender, Melissa, Neroli, Orange, Palmarosa, Rosemary, Rosewood, Sandalwood, Ylang Ylang

Therapeutic properties

* antidepressant
* antiseptic
* antispasmodic
* deodorant

* digestive
* nervine
* stomachic
* tonic

Therapeutic uses

* **Digestive system**   dyspepsia, flatulence, indigestion
* **Nervous system**   nervous exhaustion, insomnia, stress-related conditions
* **Skin care**   acne and oily skins, excessive perspiration

Psychological profile: Petitgrain is helpful for anger, confusion, disappointment, emotional shock, introversion, irrationality, mental fatigue, overactive mind, pessimism, rigidity and sadness.

Summary

Safety data

Petitgrain has no known hazards.

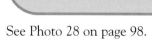

See Photo 28 on page 98.

Pine

Pine is one of the most effective oils in helping respiratory infections, sinus and bronchial congestion.

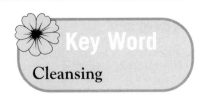

Key Word

Cleansing

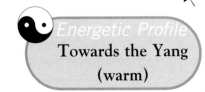

Energetic Profile

Towards the Yang (warm)

Botanical name:	Pinus sylvestris
Source:	needles and cones of the tree
Method of production:	steam distillation
Aroma characteristics:	fresh, forest aroma
Odour intensity:	high
Note:	middle
Blends well with:	Cypress, Eucalyptus, Lavender, Rosemary, Teatree, Thyme

Therapeutic properties

* antiseptic
* decongestant
* deodorant
* diuretic

* expectorant
* rubefacient
* stimulant
* tonic

Therapeutic uses

* **Musculo-skeletal system**   muscular pain and stiffness
* **Nervous system**   nervous debility; mental fatigue
* **Respiratory system**   bronchitis, breathlessness, laryngitis, flu
* **Skin care**   congested skins

Psychological profile: Pine is helpful in times of weakness and general debility.

Summary

Safety data

Pine is best used in small proportions as it may irritate sensitive skins.

See Photo 29 on page 98.

Rose

Rose is a superb oil; it is effective for skin care and has an affinity for the female reproductive system. It also has a pronounced effect on the circulatory, digestive and nervous systems.

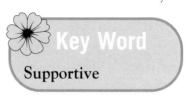

Key Word

Supportive

Botanical name:	Rosa damascena (damask rose)
	Rosa centifolia (cabbage rose)
Plant origin:	fresh petals of flowers of the shrub/plant
Method of extraction:	solvent extraction/water or steam distillation
Aroma characteristics:	rose otto has a sweet and mellow aroma with a hint of vanilla; rose absolute has a deep, rich and sweet honey-rose aroma
Odour intensity:	very high
Note:	base
Blends well with:	Bergamot, the Chamomiles, Clary Sage, Cypress, Geranium, Jasmine, Lavender, Mandarin, Neroli, Orange, Palmarosa, Patchouli, Sandalwood

Energetic Profile

Towards the Yin (cool)

Therapeutic properties

* antidepressant
* antiseptic
* antispasmodic
* antiviral
* aphrodisiac
* astringent
* bactericidal
* depurative

* emmenagogue
* haemostatic
* hepatic
* laxative
* sedative
* stomachic
* tonic (heart, liver, stomach, uterus)

Therapeutic uses

* **Circulatory system**   poor circulation, palpitations
* **Digestive system**   liver congestion
* **Endocrine system**   menstrual problems, pre-menstrual syndrome, uterine disorders
* **Nervous system**   depression, insomnia, nervous tension, stress-related problems
* **Respiratory system**   asthma, coughs, hay fever
* **Skin care**   all skin types especially dry, ageing and sensitive skins

Psychological profile: Rose is helpful for bereavement and grief, emotional trauma, insecurity, lack of confidence, lack of self-worth, melancholia and nervous tension.

Summary

Safety data

Rose has no known hazards.

See Photo 30 on page 98.

Rosemary

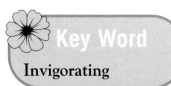

Key Word

Invigorating

Rosemary is a physical and mental stimulant that is also useful for a wide range of nervous, circulatory, muscular and digestive disorders.

Botanical name:	Rosmarinus officinalis	
Plant origin:	flowers/leaves of the herb	
Method of extraction:	steam distillation	
Aroma characteristics:	strong, herbal aroma with a clear, warm and penetrating note, camphor undertone	
Odour intensity:	high	
Note:	middle	

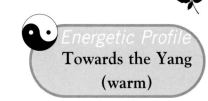

Energetic Profile
Towards the Yang (warm)

Therapeutic properties

* analgesic
* antirheumatic
* antiseptic
* antispasmodic
* astringent
* carminative
* cephalic
* cytophylactic
* digestive
* diuretic

* emmenagogue
* hepatic
* hypertensive
* nervine
* rubefacent
* stimulant (circulatory, adrenal)
* stomachic
* tonic
* vulnerary

Therapeutic uses

* **Circulatory system**   poor circulation
* **Immune system**   colds, flu
* **Lymphatic system**   fluid retention

* **Musculo-skeletal system**   muscular aches and pains, joint pain
* **Nervous system**   debility, headaches, mental fatigue, nervous exhaustion
* **Respiratory system**   asthma, bronchitis, sinusitis
* **Skin care**   especially effective for oily skin and scalp disorders

Psychological profile (uplifting and energising to the mind): Rosemary is helpful for anguish, anxiety, confusion, depression, doubt, emotional numbness and nervous debility.

Summary

Safety data

Rosemary is best avoided during pregnancy. Due to its highly stimulating actions it is best avoided by epilepsy sufferers and those with high blood pressure.

See Photo 31 on page 98.

Rosewood

Rosewood is a mild and safe choice in skin care and is also a very effective immune stimulant.

Key Word

Enlivening

Botanical name:	Aniba rosaeodora
Source:	wood chippings of the tree
Method of production:	steam distillation
Aroma characteristics:	sweet, woody, floral with a hint of spice
Odour intensity:	medium
Note:	middle
Blends well with:	Bergamot, Frankincense, Geranium, Palmarosa, Patchouli, Petitgrain, Rose, Rosemary, Sandalwood, Vetivert

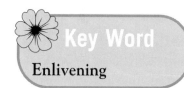

Energetic Profile
Towards the Yang (warm)

Therapeutic properties

* analgesic
* antidepressant
* antiseptic
* bactericidal
* cephalic

* deodorant
* insecticide
* stimulant
* tonic

Therapeutic uses

* **Nervous system**   headaches, nervousness and stress

* **Respiratory system**   viruses, sore throats, ticklish coughs

* **Skin care**   all skin types for cell regeneration especially the dry, sensitive and inflamed skins

Psychological profile: Rosewood is helpful for emotional instability, mood swings, nervous tension and when feeling weary and overburdened with worry.

Summary

Safety data

Rosewood appears to have no known hazards.

See Photo 32 on page 99.

Sandalwood

Sandalwood is a very subtle oil, however, it has very powerful effects on the skin and the respiratory system. It is also a valuable antidepressant and an aid to stress-related conditions, especially when associated with anxiety.

Key Word

Supportive

Botanical name:	Santalum album
Plant origin:	roots and heartwood of the tree
Method of extraction:	water or steam distillation
Aroma characteristics:	very subtle, woody and exotic aroma
Odour intensity:	medium
Note:	base note

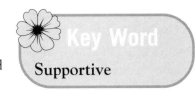

Energetic Profile

Towards the Yin (cool)

Therapeutic properties

* antidepressant
* antiseptic
* antispasmodic
* aphrodisiac
* astringent
* bactericidal

* carminative
* diuretic
* expectorant
* sedative
* tonic

Therapeutic uses

* **Digestive system**   diarrhoea, nausea

* **Immune system**   colds, flu, infections

* **Lymphatic system**   cellulite

* **Nervous system**   anxiety, depression, insomnia, nervous tension, stress-related problems

* **Respiratory system**   bronchitis, catarrh, cough, laryngitis, sore throats

* **Skin care**   effective for dry, dehydrated, oily skins and acne

* **Urinary system**   cystitis

Psychological profile: Sandalwood is helpful for apprehension, emotional exhaustion, insecurity, fear, lack of courage, nervous tension, sensitivity, shyness, tearfulness, timidity and weakness of spirit.

Summary

Safety data

Sandalwood has no known hazards.

See Photo 33 on page 99.

Tangerine

Tangerine is a gentle refreshing oil that is a useful choice for mild stress-related conditions and is useful during pregnancy.

Key Word

Revitalising

Botanical name:	Citrus reticulata
Source:	outer peel of the fruit
Method of production:	cold expression
Aroma characteristics:	light, sweet and tangy
Odour intensity:	low to medium
Note:	top
Blends well with:	Basil, Bergamot, the Chamomiles, Clary Sage, Frankincense, Geranium, Grapefruit, Lavender, Lemon, Neroli, Orange, Rose

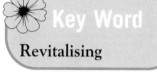

Energetic Profile
**Towards the Yin
(cool)**

Therapeutic properties

* antiseptic

* antispasmodic

* cytophylactic

* sedative

* stomachic

* tonic

Therapeutic uses

* **Digestive system**   flatulence, constipation

* **Endocrine system**   pregnancy

* **Musculo-skeletal system**   tired and aching limbs

* **Nervous system**   anxiety, depression, nervous tension, stress-related problems

* **Skin care**   all skin types; particularly effective on stretch marks and scarring

Psychological profile: Tangerine is helpful for anxiety, dejection, dwelling on the past, feelings of emptiness, grief, nervous tension, over-excitability, restlessness and shyness.

Summary

Safety data

May be phototoxic, therefore it is best to avoid exposure to strong sunlight/ultra-violet light for at least 12 hours following treatment.

See Photo 34 on page 99.

Teatree

The effects of Teatree are diverse in that it is a very effective antiseptic in skin care and with respiratory ailments. Its key quality is in strengthening the immune system.

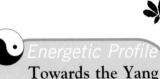

Key Word

Clarifying

Botanical name:	Melaleuca alternifolia
Source:	leaves and twigs of the tree
Method of extraction:	steam or water distillation
Aroma characteristics:	strong antiseptic aroma
Odour intensity:	very high
Note:	top
Blends well with:	Eucalyptus, Ginger, Lavender, Lemon, Mandarin, Orange, Rosemary, Thyme

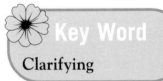

Energetic Profile
Towards the Yang (warm)

Therapeutic properties

* antibiotic
* antiseptic
* antiviral
* bactericidal
* expectorant
* fungicidal
* stimulant
* vulnerary

Therapeutic uses

* **Immune system**   colds, flu, infections
* **Respiratory system**   asthma, bronchitis, catarrh, coughs, sinusitis
* **Skin care**   oily skins
* **Urinary system**   cystitis, thrush

Psychological profile (psychic protector): Teatree is useful for fear, hypochondria, hysteria, negativity and shock.

Summary

Safety data

Teatree may cause irritation and sensitisation to some skins.

See Photo 35 on page 99.

Thyme (Common or Sweet)

Thyme is a very strong antiseptic, very effective on the respiratory and genito-urinary systems.

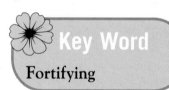

Key Word

Fortifying

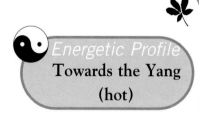

Energetic Profile

Towards the Yang (hot)

Botanical name:	Thymus vulgaris
Source:	fresh or partially dried leaves and flowering tops of herb
Method of production:	steam or water distillation
Aroma:	sweet, herbaceous and warming
Odour intensity:	high
Note:	top to middle
Blends well with:	Bergamot, the Chamomiles, Juniper, Lemon, Mandarin, Melissa, Rosemary, Teatree

Therapeutic properties

* antibiotic
* antirheumatic
* antiseptic
* antispasmodic
* antiviral
* carminative
* diuretic
* emmenagogue

* expectorant
* hypertensive
* insecticidal
* nervine
* rubefacient
* stimulates leucocytosis (production of white blood cells)

Therapeutic uses

* **Circulatory system**   poor circulation
* **Lymphatic system**   accumulation of toxins
* **Digestive system**   diarrhoea, dyspepsia, flatulence, intestinal cramps
* **Immune system**   colds
* **Nervous system**   nervous exhaustion, mental and physical fatigue
* **Respiratory system**   coughs, sore throats, tonsillitis, laryngitis, pharyngitis, whooping cough and asthma
* **Skin care**   abscesses, boils, cuts and skin infections

Psychological profile: Thyme is useful for anxiety, lack of direction, mental and psychic blockages, mental debility, mental weakness and worry.

Summary

Safety data

* Thyme is one of the strongest antiseptics and therefore should be used with care and in moderation.
* Avoid use during pregnancy or in cases of high blood pressure.
* There are a number of chemotypes of thyme available; only a few are recommended for therapeutic use.
* Red thyme contains higher proportions of the toxic chemical constituents phenols, which may cause skin irritation and sensitisation.
* White thyme is a redistillation of Red Thyme and is often adulterated.
* The oil labelled as Sweet Thyme is preferable for use in aromatherapy as it contains higher proportions of the more gentle constituents such as geraniol and linalol.

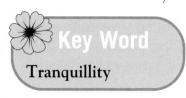

Vetivert

Vetivert is associated with inner harmony and is therefore an excellent choice for stress relief and nervous tension.

Botanical name:	Vetiveria zizanioides
Source:	dried roots and rootlets of the tall perennial grass
Method of production:	steam distillation
Aroma characteristics:	deep, earthy and smoky
Odour intensity:	high
Note:	base
Blends well with:	Benzoin, Bergamot, Frankincense, Geranium, Grapefruit, Jasmine, Lavender, Patchouli, Rose, Rosewood, Sandalwood, Ylang Ylang

Therapeutic properties

* antiseptic
* antispasmodic
* aphrodisiac
* depurative
* nervine
* rubefacient
* sedative
* tonic

Therapeutic uses

* **Musculo-skeletal system** muscular aches and pains, rheumatism, arthritis
* **Nervous system** nervous debility, stress-related problems
* **Skin care** all skin types; particularly effective on mature, dry or irritated skins

Psychological profile: Vetivert is helpful for an overactive mind, insecurity and over-sensitivity.

Summary

Safety data

Vetivert is non-toxic and non-irritant.

See Photo 36 on page 100.

Ylang Ylang

Ylang Ylang is a real comforter in times of stress; it is a very valuable antidepressant and can help to instil confidence.

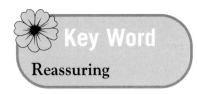

Key Word

Reassuring

Botanical name:	Cananga odorata
Plant origin:	freshly picked fragrant flowers of the small tropical tree
Method of extraction:	steam or water distillation (the first distillate is called Ylang Ylang Extra, the further successive distillates are called Ylang Ylang 1, 2, and 3)
Aroma characteristics:	very sweet heavy, floral and exotic aroma, with a musky undertone
Odour intensity:	high
Note:	base

Energetic Profile

Towards the Yin (cool)

Therapeutic properties

* antidepressant
* antiseptic
* aphrodisiac
* euphoric
* hypotensive
* nervine
* regulator (hormonal and sebum)
* sedative (nervous)
* stimulant (circulatory)
* tonic (uterine)

Therapeutic uses

* **Circulatory system** high blood pressure
* **Hormonal system** hormonal problems
* **Nervous system** anxiety, depression, insomnia, nervous tension, stress-related problems
* **Skin care** oily and dry skins

Psychological profile (confidence booster): Ylang Ylang is useful for anger, insecurity, fear, frustration, panic, introversion, lack of confidence, jealousy, sensitivity and stubbornness.

Summary

Safety data

Ylang Ylang may cause sensitisation in some skins. Use in low concentrations as its heady aroma may cause headaches and nausea.

See Photo 37 on page 100.

Complete the following tables by identifying the following information:

Task

* the common name of the essential oil
* the origin of the oil (i.e. the part of the plant from which it is produced)
* the method of production
* list five known properties attributed to this oil.

Botanical name	Common name of essential oil	Source	Method of production	Properties
Citrus bergamia				
Rose dameascena				
Rosemarinus officinalis				
Santalum album				

✳ Table 1: The Essential Oils ✳

Botanical name	Common name of essential oil	Source	Method of production	Properties
Cananga odorata				
Piper nigrum				
Anthemis nobilis				
Salvia sclarea				

* Table 1: Continued *

Botanical name	Common name of essential oil	Source	Method of production	Properties
Eucalyptus globulus				
Botswellia carteri				
Pelargonium graveolens				
Juniperus communis				

* Table 1: Continued *

Botanical name	Common name of essential oil	Source	Method of production	Properties
Lavendula officinalis				
Citrus limonum				
Origanum majorana				
Mentha piperita				

* Table 1: Continued *

Self-assessment Questions

1. Why is it often said that essential oils contain the life force of the plant?

----

2. Why is it important to be able to recognise the botanical name of a plant in connection with an essential oil?

----

3. Define the following terms used to describe the therapeutic properties of essential oils:

   i)   analgesic

----

   ii) antispasmodic

----

   iii) rubefacient

----

   iv) febrifuge

----

   v) cytophylactic

----

   vi) carminative

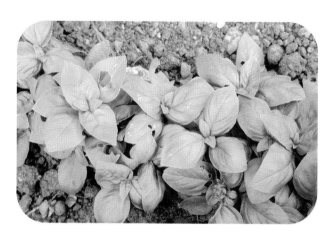

❈ Photo 1: Basil (sweet) ❈

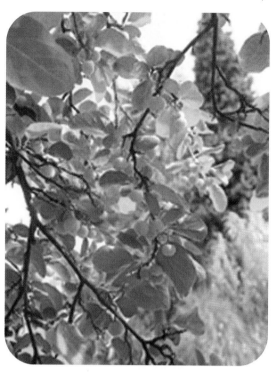

❈ Photo 2: Benzoin ❈

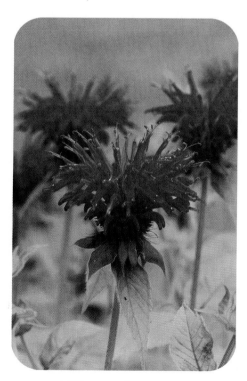

❈ Photo 3: Bergamot ❈

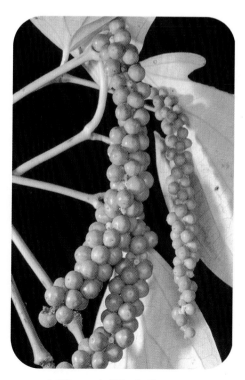

❈ Photo 4: Black Pepper ❈

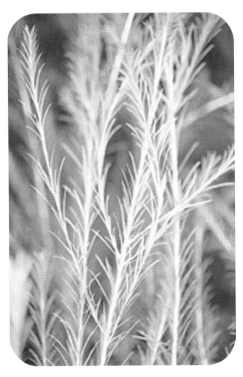

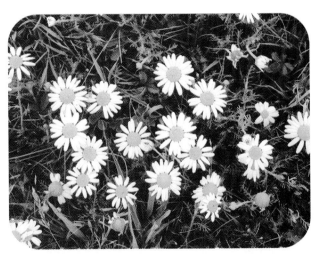

✳ Photo 6: Roman Chamomile, German/Blue Chamomile and Moroccan Chamomile ✳

✳ Photo 5: Cajeput ✳

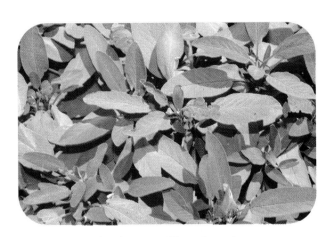

✳ Photo 7: Clary Sage ✳

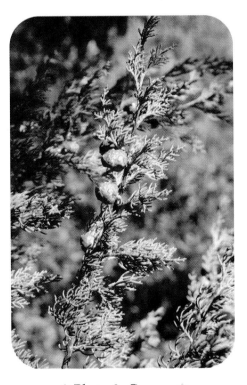

✳ Photo 8: Cypress ✳

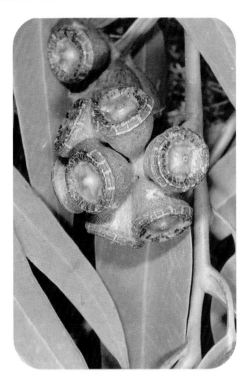

※ Photo 9: Eucalyptus ※

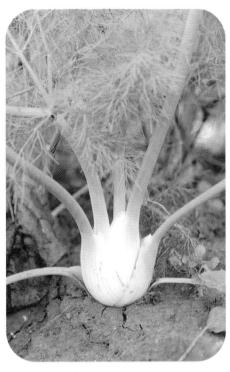

※ Photo 10: Fennel ※

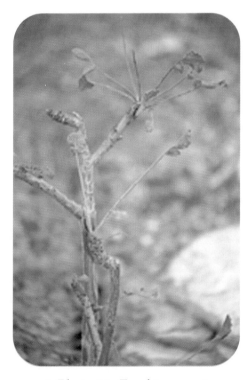

※ Photo 11: Frankincense ※

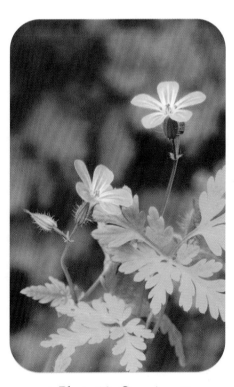

※ Photo 12: Geranium ※

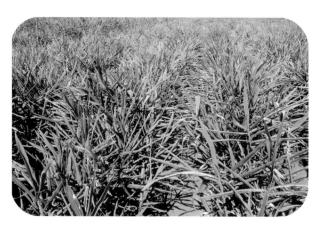

❋ Photo 13: Ginger ❋

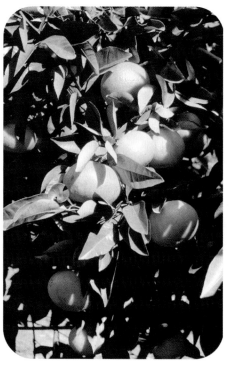

❋ Photo 14: Grapefruit ❋

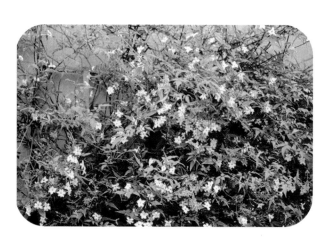

❋ Photo 15: Jasmine ❋

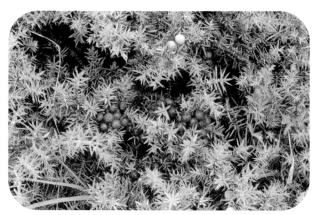

❋ Photo 16: Juniper ❋

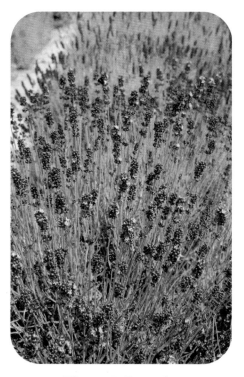

* Photo 17: Lavender *

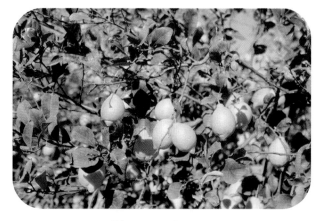

* Photo 18: Lemon *

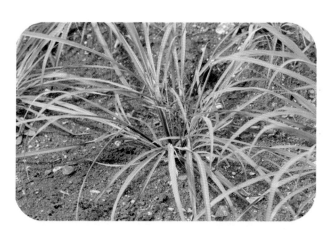

* Photo 19: Lemongrass *

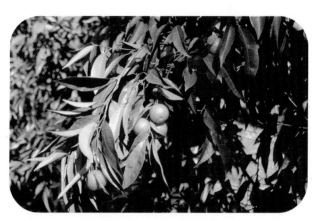

* Photo 20: Mandarin *

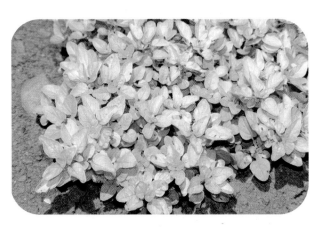

✳ Photo 21: Marjoram (Sweet) ✳

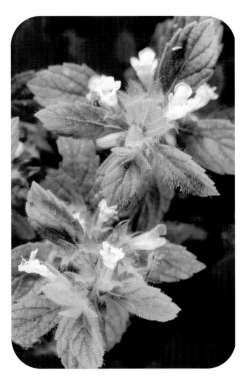

✳ Photo 22: Melissa ✳

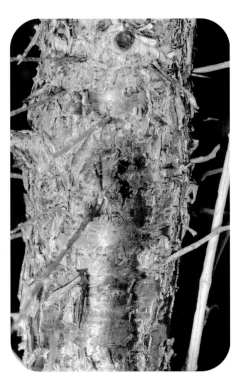

✳ Photo 23: Myrrh ✳

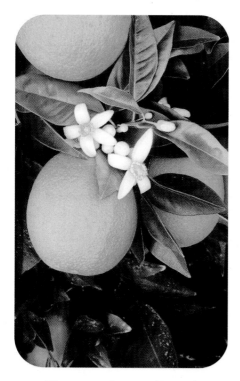

❋ Photo 24: Orange (Sweet) ❋

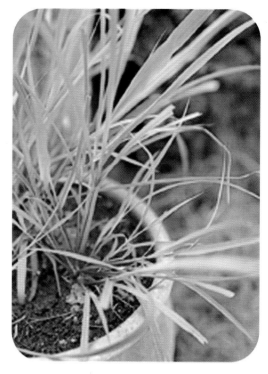

❋ Photo 25: Palmarosa ❋

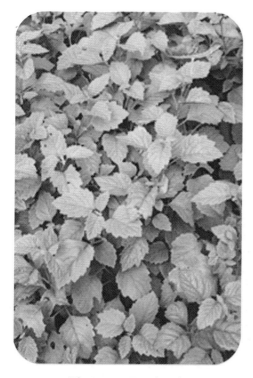

❋ Photo 26: Patchouli ❋

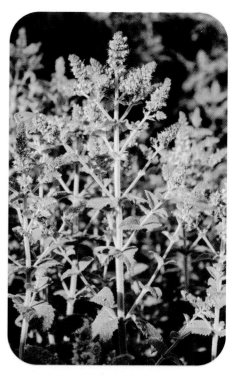

❋ Photo 27: Peppermint ❋

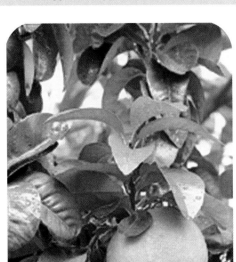

* Photo 28: Petitgrain and Neroli oil *

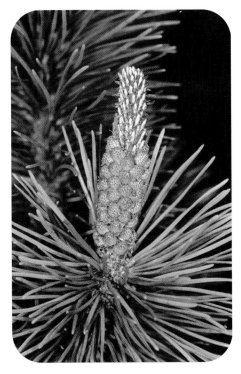

* Photo 29: Pine *

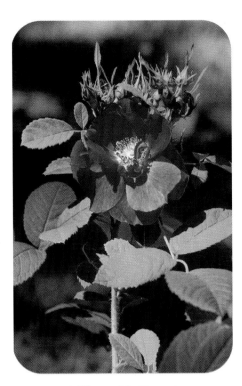

* Photo 30: Rose *

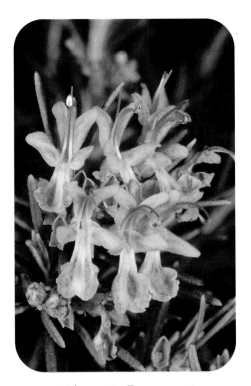

* Photo 31: Rosemary *

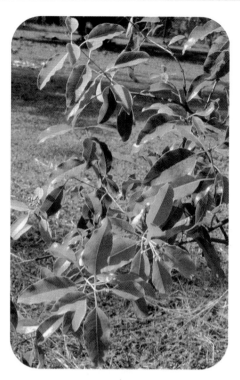

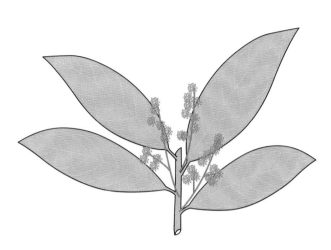

❋ Photo 32: Rosewood ❋

❋ Photo 33: Sandalwood ❋

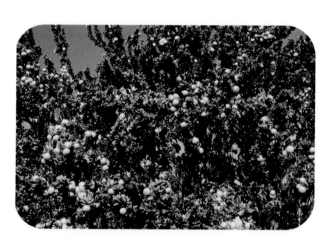

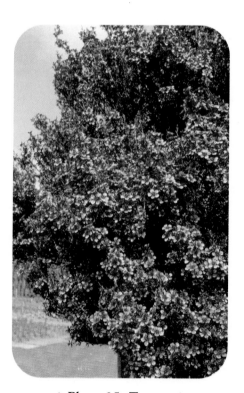

❋ Photo 34: Tangerine ❋

❋ Photo 35: Teatree ❋

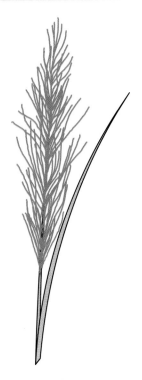

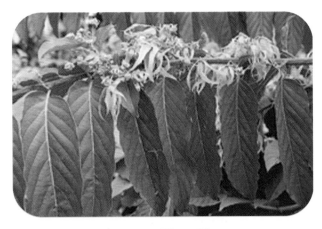

✳ Photo 37: Ylang Ylang ✳

✳ Photo 36: Vetivert ✳

CHAPTER 5

Basic Chemistry for Aromatherapy

A typical essential oil comprises over 100 chemical compounds, and therefore has an extremely complex chemical structure. Many of the chemical compounds contained within essential oils are hard to detect and some are present only in minute quantities, making chemistry of essential oils a complex subject to study.

The chemical make-up of an essential oil generally reflects its therapeutic effects and toxicology; in this chapter we will consider the basics of chemistry that are relevant to an aromatherapist.

✻ A competent aromatherapist needs a basic knowledge of chemistry, in order to understand the therapeutic properties of essential oils, along with their potential hazards.

Objectives

By the end of this chapter you will be able to relate the following knowledge to your work as an aromatherapist:

✻ the basic principles of organic chemistry

✻ the classifications of essential oil compounds

✻ examples of common chemical constituents of essential oils

✻ basic chemical structures in relation to essential oils

✻ common analytical techniques used in the identification of the chemical constituents of an essential oil.

Before looking at the individual compounds that make up an essential oil, it is important to consider the *biosynthesis* of the plant, which is the term used to describe the building up of complex organic compounds, from which the essential oil is derived.

Within their structures, green plants have specialised mechanisms that are capable of synthesising complex carbohydrates from simple starting materials such as hydrogen, carbon and oxygen.

Chemical synthesis requires energy. The energy required by plants to carry out these tasks comes entirely from the sun; this process is known as *photosynthesis*.

Photosynthesis is the process by which a plant, under the influence of sunlight, can build up carbohydrates from the carbon dioxide of the atmosphere and hydrogen from the water in the soil.

The Biosynthesis Pathway of Essential Oils

The biochemical steps by which larger complex organic compounds are synthesised from carbohydrates is as follows:

* The pathway originates in plants where carbon dioxide and oxygen are converted into a six-carbon sugar Glucose ($C_6H_{12}O_6$).

* Glucose is then split into two three-carbon compounds through an oxidation reaction in which hydrogen atoms are lost. This result is a compound called pyruvic acid ($C_3H_4O_3$).

* Pyruvic acid is then further broken down to acetic acid ($C_2H_4O_2$).

Acetic acid molecules are very important to the synthesis of essential oils as they are converted via a series of condensation (removal of H_2O) and reduction reactions to a compound called mevalonic acid.

Mevalonic acid has been found to be the root source of many molecular compounds found in essential oils.

Mevalonic acid is then converted into a compound known as a *terpene*. This is a hydrocarbon compound, which, through a series of reduction and oxidation reactions, synthesises a plethora of aromatic carbohydrates. These are the bulk of the compounds found in essential oils.

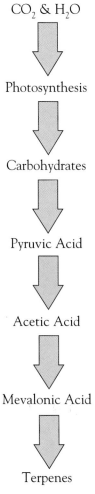

CO$_2$ & H$_2$O

Photosynthesis

Carbohydrates

Pyruvic Acid

Acetic Acid

Mevalonic Acid

Terpenes

* **Figure 3: Flow chart** *

> ## Key Note
>
> It is important for aromatherapists to realise that the final molecular content of an essential oil is very much dependent on the source and availability of its original ingredients, such as carbon dioxide, water and light, as well as the environment within the plant itself.

Basic Principles of Organic Chemistry

Aromatherapists are the 'end users' of the essential oils, but it is important to appreciate that before they undertake their work the plant has been produced from very simple building blocks such as light, carbon dioxide and water.

Plants have an amazing ability to synthesise chemical substances, and as mentioned above, essential oil extracted from plant materials can contain several hundred chemical constituents. It is therefore appropriate to consider the basic chemistry of carbon (C), as carbon dioxide (CO_2) is the base material used to construct all the body of plants. Carbon is a very useful element, and without it the world would be a very different place; it is at the heart of all that we are and all of the materials around us.

Essential oils are *organic* compounds, which means that they all contain the element carbon. Hydrogen, carbon and oxygen are the building blocks of essential oils, and each of these elements is itself made up of atoms and molecules – the building blocks of the universe:

⁎ atoms are the smallest units of any element

⁎ molecules are the smallest units of a compound.

Compounds are formed when atoms are bonded, that is, they are joined together. There are therefore two different classifications of essential oil compounds:

⁎ **Hydrocarbons**   the first major category of compounds; these contain molecules of hydrogen and carbon only and are classified as *Terpenes*.

⁎ **Oxygenated compounds**   the second major category of compounds; these contain hydrogen, carbon and also oxygen, and are classified under different chemical types such as *Acids*, *Alcohols*, *Aldehydes*, *Esters*, *Ketones*, *Lactones*, *Oxides* and *Phenols*.

Note: the compounds listed above are found throughout nature and are not exclusive to the world of aromatherapy and essential oils.

Chemical Structure of Essential Oils

There are two main building blocks for the chemical structure of essential oils.

٭ **Isoprene unit** these structures are made up of five carbon compounds in a branched chain; see Figure 4.

$$CH_2 = C - CH_2 - CH_2 - \qquad CH_2$$

٭ **Figure 4: Isoprene unit** ٭

٭ **Aromatic rings** another feature of carbon chemistry is the ability to form rings. Carbon atoms do not always join together in a branched chain, sometimes they join together in a ring, forming what is known as an aromatic ring. As the chain length increases, the potential to form rings increases. Rings can form from three carbon atoms but most are comprised of five or six atoms.

٭ **Figure 5: Aromatic ring** ٭

Organic chemistry (the chemistry of compounds containing carbon) also utilises oxygen (O), nitrogen (N), sulphur (S) as basic molecular building blocks. It is not surprising that from these basic elements it is possible to build a vast array of compounds.

Terpenes

These contain less than the maximum number of hydrogen atoms, and are referred to as 'unsaturated'. They are based on the isoprene unit, which is a five-carbon compound.

There are two main types of terpene of interest to an aromatherapist:

٭ **Monoterpenes** all molecules of monoterpenes contain ten carbon units, as they are made up of two isoprene units. Common examples of monoterpenes include *limonene* (found in Lemon, Bergamot, Neroli and Orange), and *pinene* (found in Cypress and Eucalyptus).

Monoterpenes are found in practically all essential oils. They have weak, uninteresting odours, are very volatile and readily oxidise.

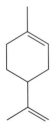

٭ **Figure 6: Limonene (monoterpene)** ٭

٭ **Sesquiterpenes** atoms of sesquiterpenes contain 15 carbon atoms and are therefore made up of three isoprene units. The prefix 'sesqui' means 'one and a half'. Sesquiterpenes are a less common chemical component of essential oils. They have a strong odour and can have an important influence on the fragrance of an essential oil. Common examples of sesquiterpenes include *chamazulene* (found in the Chamomiles), *bisabolene* (found in Black Pepper and Lemon), and *caryophyllene* (found in Lavender, Marjoram and Clary Sage).

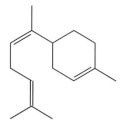

❋ Figure 7: Bisabolene (sesquiterpene) ❋

Oxygenated Compounds

Key Note

It is important to remember that it is the odour of oxygenated compounds and sesquiterpenes that determine the fragrance characteristics of essential oils.

Acids

This category of organic compounds is a rare component of essential oils. Structurally they are based on the carboxyl group and have the chemical grouping COOH.

Acids have a low volatility rate. Common examples of acids found in essential oils include *benzoic* acid in Benzoin, and *geranic* acid in Geranium.

❋ Figure 8: Benzoic acid ❋

Alcohols

These are based on monoterpenes and therefore contain ten carbon atoms. They contain the chemical functional group OH. They are referred to as terpene derivatives and are classified on the basis of which type of terpene was involved in their production:

❋ **Monoterpenic alcohols**   these are the most common type of alcohols found in essential oils. Examples include *linalool* (found in Rosewood), and *geraniol* (found in Geranium).

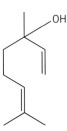

* Figure 9: Linalool (monoterpenic alcohol) *

* **Sesquiterpenic alcohols** these are not so common and are based on the sesquiterpenes as the name suggests. A common example of a sesquiterpenic alcohol is *santalol* (found in Sandalwood).

Aldehydes

This category of organic compounds is a common essential oil component, and is based on the carbonyl group (C = O). Aldehydes have a slightly fruity odour when the odour is smelt on its own. Some aldehydes are used as skin irritants and sensitisers. Common examples of aldehydes in essential oils include *citronellol* (found in Citronella), and *citral* (found in Lemongrass).

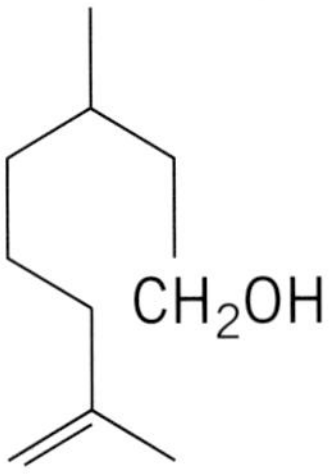

* Figure 10: Citronellol (aldehyde) *

Esters

These are very important constituents of essential oils. They are produced from the corresponding terpene alcohol and an organic acid, and are based on the carboxyl group (COOH).

The highest levels of esters are produced on the full bloom of the flower or the maturity of the fruit or plant. For example, bergamot: as the fruit begins to ripen, linalool is converted to linalyl acetate.

Common examples of esters found in essential oils include *linalyl acetate* (found in Bergamot, Clary Sage and Lavender), and *geranyl acetate* (found in Sweet Marjoram).

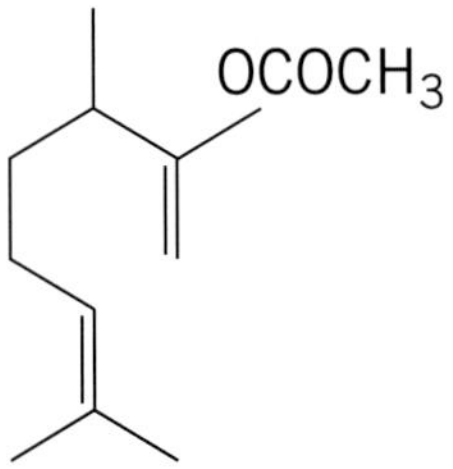

* Figure 11: Linalyl acetate (ester) *

Ketones

These are potentially toxic compounds and are similar in structure to aldehydes, being based on the carbonyl group (C = O).

Common examples of ketones found in essential oils include *fenchone* (found in Fennel), and *camphor* (found in Rosemary).

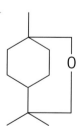

* **Figure 12: Camphor (ketone)** *

Lactones

These are found mainly in expressed oils. A sub-group of lactones called furocoumarins is known as photo-sensitisers, and *bergaptene* is the most common molecular example.

* **Figure 13: Bergaptene (furocoumarin-lactone)** *

Oxides

These chemical compounds are rarely found in essential oils. They tend to be non-hazardous, and their chemical structure is such that the oxygen atom in the molecule is situated between two carbon atoms: C—O—C.

A common example of an oxide found in essential oils is *cineole*; in its most common form it is known as 1,8 cineole (found in Eucalyptus).

* **Figure 14: 1,8 cineole (oxide)** *

Phenols

This category of aromatic molecules is similar to the alcohols in that they have an —OH group. In phenols, however, the OH group attaches itself to carbon in an aromatic ring.

The significance of the OH group is that it makes the phenol molecule very reactive, which explains why essential oils containing a high proportion of phenols can be irritating to the skin.

Common examples of essential oils containing phenols include: *thymol* (found in Thyme), *cavacrol* (found in Thyme), and *eugenol* (found in Clove, Cinnamon Leaf and Black Pepper).

✳ **Figure 15: Thymol** ✳

Summary

The two most important points are that carbon is at the heart of all essential oils, and that essential oils are made by living plants. A vast array of different compounds can be made by adding carbon atoms together, and this is increased further when we add other atoms like oxygen. The size of a molecule, its shape and the concentration of chemical constituents within the oil will therefore confer its individual and collective properties.

Chemical Compounds and Therapeutic Properties of Essential Oils

Different essential oils have varying therapeutic properties according to their molecular content.

All chemical compounds have widely varying properties and therefore it is virtually impossible to generalise about the therapeutic properties based only on the properties of the known chemical constituents, as the whole essential oil is more active than its principal constituents.

It is also possible that minor or trace constituents may contribute to the therapeutic properties more than the major constituents.

It can therefore be concluded that the combination *and* concentration of its chemical constituents reflect an essential oil's individual and collective properties.

Chemotypes

The same plant grown in different regions and under different conditions can produce essential oils of widely diverse characteristics. Variations in the chemical constituents of the oil occur and are known as *chemotypes*. The word 'chemotype' is also used to indicate oils of different chemical composition, even though they are obtained from plants that are botanically identical. Chemotypes are quite common, and essential oils will naturally vary from season to season due to the following factors:

* condition and type of soil in which the plant is grown
* region or country from which the oil was sourced
* method of extraction
* climate and conditions such as altitude.

Key Note

Due to the variations in climate and soil, the natural chemistry of an essential oil will not be present in exactly the same proportions at each distillation. This explains why essential oils vary from batch to batch.

Techniques used in Essential Oil Analysis

It is generally accepted that the quality and 'wholeness' of an essential oil used in aromatherapy is fundamental to its therapeutic efficacy. This may be due to a number of factors:

* minor trace constituents may have therapeutic benefits

* the total benefit conferred by the whole oil is greater than the sum of its individual components

* little is known about the pharmacological actions of *all* the constituents present within an essential oil

* it is difficult to produce a synthetic, simpler mixture of oils until all the individual and additive effects can be scientifically documented.

Unfortunately, there is no perfect single, analytical technique capable of identifying all the constituents chemically. However, if a reputable analytical laboratory is employed using validated methods, it is possible to 'fingerprint' an oil and compare it to a known reference.

Gas Liquid Chromatography

The technique commonly used in essential oils analysis is *Gas Liquid Chromatography* (GLC), known simply as GC. The term chromatography simply means the separation of the components of a mixture.

A Russian botanist called Michael Tswett (1872–1919) was the grandfather of modern chromatography. He discovered basic principles of column chromatography when separating plant pigments. The various pigments were separated into coloured bands, hence the name chromatography ('chromo' is Greek for colour).

Apparatus

In its most basic form, the GC apparatus comprises the following components:

* the column (typically 1–60 metres long), which is coated with a thin film of liquid

* an oven that houses the column and is capable of working within the temperature range 40–450 °C

* an injection port (the means of placing the essential oil into the column)

* a detector (the means of 'seeing' the products of the GC separation)

* a syringe (capable of injecting very small quantities, typically 0.2–5 µl).

Method

* A small amount of essential oil is injected into the port to be analysed. The amount of time taken for each chemical compound to emerge at the other end of the column (known as the retention time) is different, due to the fact that all chemical components are of different molecular size.

* The interaction of the sample components with the gas phase and the liquid phase achieves the separation.

* The quantity of each chemical component is then analysed by the detector and a peak is shown on the trace, which relates proportionally to its quantity.

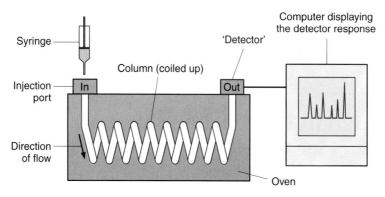

* **Figure 16: Gas Chromatograph** *

The retention time of a given component is a character of that component, and can be used to assign its identity, provided that a pure single component sample is also analysed. However, if the individual identity is not known, the analysis can be carried out and the whole chromatogram can be compared to a reference oil known to be of high quality. This process forms the basis of fingerprinting an essential oil.

The choice of detector used will influence the quality of the data collected, as some detectors can produce accurate quantitative data and others can identify the individual chemicals. Examples of two types of detector commonly used are:

* flame ionisation detector (FID)

* mass spectrometer.

The latest carbon-13 NMR spectroscopy provides an alternative method of essential oil analysis. The efficient visual spacing of the signals enables essential oil samples to be analysed without the preliminary separation of their components.

An excellent reference is *Essential Oil Analysis by Capillary Gas Chromatography and Carbon-13 NMR Spectroscopy* 2nd Edition (ISBN 0-471-96314-3), which includes qualitative and quantitative analysis data of 60 commercially important essential oils and 188 of the most important chemical constituents found in essential oils.

Because essential oils contain several chemical functional groups and have high carbon numbers, they produce complex chromatograms.

Key Note

Gas Chromatography is not a guaranteed test of purity, but is a comparative test; each batch tested is compared to a known reference, which is the 'standard'. However, it is possible to highlight adulterants that are not evident on the 'standard'.

Essential Oils and a Question of Purity

It is generally accepted that in aromatherapy wholeness and quality of essential oils are of paramount importance.

In other trades that use essential oils, such as the perfumery industry, standardisation is important, as essential oils are adjusted to suit the desired aromas.

In aromatherapy, however, it is important to preserve wholeness to guard against its natural synergy, as the components that make up an essential oil co-operate to produce its healing effects.

When single active compounds are removed from an essential oil, not only is the synergy diminished but also isolated components may need greater care when used alone and may produce side effects, which seemed to be quenched when used in the whole oil.

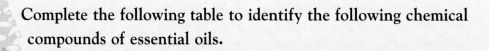

Complete the following table to identify the following chemical compounds of essential oils.

Task

Chemical compounds	Description
	Based on the carboxyl group (COOH). Rare components of essential oil; have a low volatility rate.
	Contain ten carbon atoms and the chemical functional group OH. Are referred to as terpene derivatives.
	Based on the carboxyl group (C = O). Commonly found as essential oil components. Some may be skin irritants and sensitisers.
	Produced from the corresponding terpene alcohol and organic acid. Based on carboxyl group (COOH). Very important constituents of essential oils.
	Based on carbonyl group (C—O), potentially toxic compounds. Similar in structure to aldehydes.
	Mainly found in expressed oil. Contain the sub group furocoumarins, which are photo-sensitisers.
	The structure of these compounds is that the oxygen atom in the molecule is situated between two carbon atoms C—O—C. Found rarely in essential oils.
	Contain the functional group OH, which attaches itself to a carbon in an aromatic ring. Can be irritating to the skin.
	Contain ten carbon units and are therefore made up of two isoprene units. Found in practically all essential oils.
	These compounds contain 15 carbon atoms and are made up of three isoprene units. Less common components of essential oils; have an important influence on the fragrance of an essential oil.

✳ Table 4: Chemical compounds of essential oils ✳

Self-assessment Questions

1. Name the chemical elements that represent the basic building blocks for essential oils.

----

2. State the two classifications of essential oil components, and their sub classifications.

----

3. Describe the two main chemical structures that form the main building blocks for essential oils.

----

4. What is meant by the term chemotype?

----

5. What is Gas Chromatography?

----

6. Why is it impossible to analyse all chemical constituents of an essential oil?

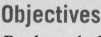

The Physiology of Aromatherapy

CHAPTER 6

In aromatherapy there are two ways in which essential oils may be absorbed into the bloodstream to have therapeutic effects: through the skin, and via the respiratory system. The effects of aromatherapy upon the body are so diverse because essential oils have three distinct modes of action:

* *they initiate chemical changes in the body when the essential oil enters the bloodstream and reacts with hormones and enzymes*
* *they have a physiological effect on the systems of the body*
* *they have a psychological effect when the odour of the oil is inhaled.*

* A competent aromatherapist needs to understand the effects of aromatherapy to appreciate the principles upon which it works.

Objectives

By the end of this chapter you will be able to relate the following knowledge to your work as an aromatherapist:

* how essential oils enter the bloodstream
* the process of olfaction
* the effects of aromatherapy on the major systems of the body.

The Absorption of Essential Oils into the Bloodstream

In aromatherapy, there are two ways in which essential oils may be absorbed into the bloodstream for therapeutic effect: through the skin and via respiration.

The way in which aromatherapy works is often subject to a degree of debate as to whether essential oils work because of their chemical constituents or because of their route of administration, such as massage.

The skin

As the skin is the largest surface area for the application of essential oils, it represents the most common route for absorbing essential oils into the bloodstream for therapeutic effect.

The skin is divided into two main layers:

* the upper, most superficial layer, the **epidermis**, which is divided into five layers: horny layer, clear layer, granular layer, prickle cell layer and the basal cell layer

* the deeper layer, **dermis**, which contains appendages such as the hair, hair follicles, sweat glands, sebaceous glands and an abundance of blood vessels that provide vital nourishment to the epidermis.

Essential oils are made up of tiny organic molecules that enable them to penetrate the skin and cross the horny layer of the epidermis, by entering the ducts of the sweat glands and hair follicles to reach the upper dermis and the capillary circulation. Essential oils are absorbed through the skin by simple diffusion, as the skin is semi-permeable and essential oils contain constituents that are primarily fat-soluble and partially water-soluble. The fat-soluble aromatic particles of the essential oil dissolve in the oily sebum produced by the sebaceous glands, and pass into the deeper layer of the skin (the dermis) where they are then carried by the blood and lymph vessels into the main bloodstream.

The rate of absorption of essential oils may be dependent on several factors:

* The composition of the oil (oils with a lower volatility rate will take longer to be absorbed).

* The viscosity of the carrier oil/s.

* The condition of the client's skin (excess fat, oedema, sluggish circulation and excess tissue toxication will slow down absorption).

Factors that can enhance the absorption of essential oils include:

* Stimulation and increased blood flow (via massage).

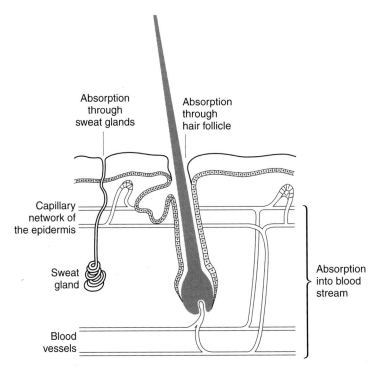

* **Figure 17: The absorption of essential oils into the skin** *

* Heat (treatment room should be comfortably warm and clients should be covered and kept warm after the massage in order to aid absorption).

* Clean skin (clients should ideally come for treatment pre-showered with all body creams and lotions removed).

* Client may also be encouraged to carry out dry skin brushing prior to an aromatherapy massage in order to remove the dead keratinised layer of the skin.

* The amount of essential oil molecules reaching the bloodstream will be greatly enhanced by encouraging the client to breathe deeply throughout an aromatherapy massage.

Key Note

The top layer of the epidermis (the horny layer) acts as a reservoir where essential oils components can continue for several hours.

Essential oils diffuse through the skin at different rates and in certain cases can take up to 90 minutes to be absorbed into the bloodstream. Much depends on the surface area to which essential oils are applied, the viscosity (thickness) of the carrier oil used and the volatility rate of the essential oils.

The rate of absorption of essential oils into the skin increases greatly if the skin is damaged. Care must therefore be taken to avoid application of essential oils to broken skin, in order to prevent skin irritation and sensitisation.

Aromatherapy can help the skin in the following ways:

* Aromatherapy massage increases the absorption rate of essential oils into the skin, which penetrate the skin due to their small molecular size.

* Essential oils can help to enhance the protective function of the skin due to the fact that many essential oils are antiseptic, antibacterial and anti-fungal; for example Lavender, Lemon, Bergamot and Teatree.

* Essential oils can help the skin's cells to regenerate; examples of this are cytophylactic oils such as Lavender and Neroli.

* Essential oils can help to calm and soothe the skin; for example Chamomile, which is anti-inflammatory.

* Essential oils can help to regulate the skin by balancing the secretion of sebum; for example Geranium can be used to help both dry and oily skins.

The respiratory system

Respiration is one of the most basic functions of the body. Through the process of gas exchange in the lungs, essential oil particles can diffuse into the bloodstream. After passing through the nose where it has been warmed, moistened and filtered, the inhaled air (carrying aromatic particles of an essential oil) continues its journey towards the lungs. It passes through the pharynx, the larynx, the trachea and into the bronchi. Within the lungs, each bronchus divides and subdivides into smaller tubes called bronchioles. Each bronchiole then divides into alveoli – these are composed of a very thin membrane of simple epithelium, only a single layer thick, so that the process of diffusion can take place.

The function of this very large expanse of film is to allow the exchange of gases between the air in the lungs and the blood in the bloodstream. Each cluster of alveoli is surrounded by a very rich network of capillaries and a moist membrane. The inhaled air carrying the essential oil particles is able to pass through these thin layers after being dissolved in the surface moisture. The capillaries surrounding the alveoli join up to form venules and arterioles, which in turn join up to form larger veins and arteries.

Therefore, any substance inhaled with the air will be involved in this complete process of gas exchange. Differing amounts of aromatic particles of essential oil will therefore be dissolved into the bloodstream from the lungs.

Key Note

The actual amount of essential oil dissolved into the bloodstream depends on the volatility and chemical structure of the oil concerned. The absorption of essential oils into the bloodstream via the respiratory system is slower and more diffusive than any other form of application, and essential oils will not build up high levels of concentration (as long as sensible proportions are used), due to the fact that the oils are constantly being removed from the bloodstream by one or more exit pathways.

The amount of essential oil absorbed into the bloodstream can be measured by analysis of exhaled breath, blood and urine samples.

Aromatherapy massage can help the respiratory systems if suitable oils are combined, which can help promote good breathing by clearing the lungs and allowing the interchange of gases to occur more efficiently.

In some cases, however, it may be more effective to use an inhalation where the physical condition would contra-indicate massage, as in the case of a client with a heavy cold. Essential oils that have an affinity for the respiratory system include:

* antiseptic oils such as Lavender, Bergamot, Lemon, Sandalwood, Juniper, Eucalyptus and Teatree, which help to prevent infections of the respiratory tract

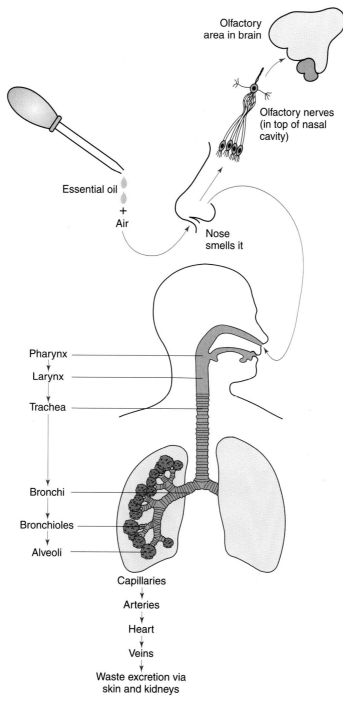

Olfactory
area in brain

Olfactory nerves
(in top of nasal
cavity)

Essential oil
+
Air

Nose
smells it

Pharynx
↓
Larynx
↓
Trachea
↓
Bronchi
↓
Bronchioles
↓
Alveoli
↓
Capillaries
↓
Arteries
↓
Heart
↓
Veins
↓
Waste excretion via
skin and kidneys

✳ **Figure 18: The journey of an essential oil** ✳

* antiviral oils such as Lavender, Teatree and Eucalyptus, which are effective in helping viral infections of the respiratory tract
* antispasmodic oils such as Clary Sage, Peppermint and Frankincense can help to calm spasms in the bronchial tubes
* expectorants that are most effective in the removal of excess phlegm incude Eucalpytus, Peppermint and Sandalwood.

The Theory of Olfaction

Olfaction is a special sense in that odour perception is transmitted directly to the brain.

The process of olfaction may be summarised as follows:

Reception

* The volatile particles of an essential oil evaporate on contact with air (some volatile molecules pervade the air and some enter the nose).
* The odiferous particles of the essential oil dissolve in the mucus that lines the inner nasal cavity, prior to their stimulation at the receptor sites.

Transmission

* The captivated aromatic molecules are picked up by the cilia, which protrude from the olfactory receptor cells (located at the top of the nasal cavity).
* The olfactory receptor cells have a long nerve fibre called an axon and an electrochemical message of the aroma is transmitted along the axons of receptor cells to join the olfactory nerves.
* The fibres of the olfactory nerves pass through the cribriform plate of the ethmoid bone in the roof of the nose to reach the olfactory bulb where the odorant signal is chemically converted before being relayed to the brain.

Perception

* Once the message reaches the olfactory bulb, the olfactory impulses pass into the olfactory tract and pass directly to the cerebral cortex where the smell is perceived.
* The temporal lobe of the brain contains the primary olfactory area, which is directly connected to the limbic area.

Key Note

Smell is the only sense that has a direct access route to the brain.

In most nerves of the body, the passing on of messages or impulses about the environment is done through the spinal cord and from there on to the brain. However, in the case of the olfactory cells, the nerve fibres pass through a bony plate at the top of the nose and connect directly with the area of the brain known as the olfactory bulb, which is situated in the cerebral cortex.

As the cilia are in direct contact with the source of smell and as the olfactory receptor cells connect directly with the brain, the sense of smell has a powerful and immediate effect on the body.

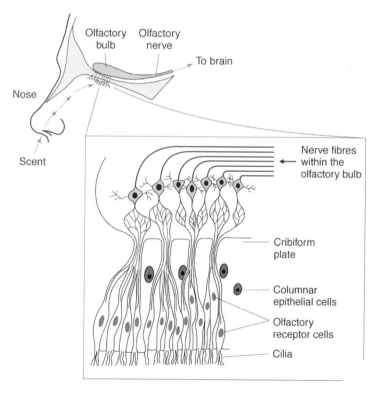

✳ Figure 19: The theory of olfaction ✳

The Limbic System

The limbic system is a v-shaped structure sitting on top of the brain stem, and includes the amalygdae, hippocampus, part of the thalamus and the hypothalamus.

The *hippocampus* is involved in memory function and is a paired organ, with one located in each temporal lobe of the brain. In relation to olfaction, the hippocampus helps us to link that odour to its 'memory bank', to determine whether it is a familiar fragrance and, if so, which related memories are brought forward into our conscious awareness. The *amygdalae* are located symmetrically in the limbic system just above the hypothalamus in the anterior tip of the temporal lobes. It is thought that the amygdala works with the *hypothalamus* to mediate emotional responses; certain odours may precipitate varied emotions from pleasure to rage and aggression.

The anterior part of the limbic system is in the olfactory cortex, which explains the intimate relationship between smells and emotions.

Another part of the limbic system, called the *septum pellicidum*, is said to be the pleasure centre. Electrical impulses applied to this part of the brain have evoked happiness in depressed persons, pain relief in cancer sufferers and intensification of sexual arousal in some people.

The limbic system receives sensory input from the olfactory, visual, auditory, balance and equilibrium systems. It processes much of this input, and channels it to the cerebral cortex. It forms connections with the brain stem below and the cerebrum above and allows for a balance and integration of emotion and reason; see Figure 20(a).

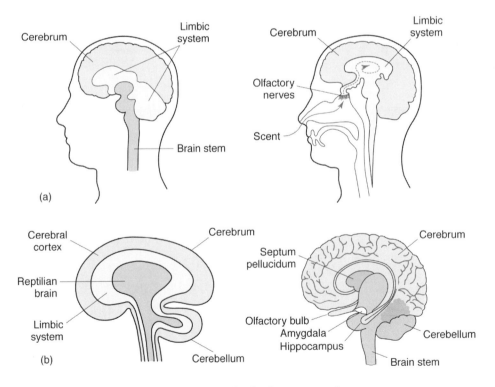

✳ Figure 20: The limbic system ✳

The limbic system has multiple connections with the thalamus, hypothalamus and pituitary gland, which is why olfactory sensory receptors can influence endocrine function.

Functionally, the limbic system is a complex structure that has approximately 34 structures and 53 pathways. It is the major seat of our emotions, and is linked to the perception of odour, sensations of pleasure and pain, emotions like rage, fear, sadness and sexual feelings.

The complexity of the limbic systems and the direct link between the olfactory receptor cells and the limbic area of the brain explain why smell can effect an emotional response and recall a memory from the past, as scent memory is longer-term than visual memory; see Figure 20(b).

The Circulatory System

The heart is a pump that constantly distributes blood to and from the lungs and all around the body in a double circuit. All chemical substances that need to be transported around the body are carried by the blood, e.g. hormones. The blood circulates around the body at a surprisingly fast speed, taking about a half minute to complete a circuit. This means that when substances such as essential oil particles are dissolved into the blood-stream, they can take effect very quickly.

Some essential oils have affinities with certain organs or systems, and will have a special effect on that organ or system when at that point in its circulating journey. The oils will be either wholly or partly deposited in any organs for which they have a special affinity; others will exercise a more general effect.

Whatever part of the essential oil is left after its therapeutic work in the body has been done, will be excreted by one path or another. It may be passed out of the body in urine or faeces, excreted through the skin as sweat or returned to the lungs to be exhaled with the breath.

How aromatherapy can help the circulatory system

Combining essential oils with aromatherapy massage techniques can help our circulatory system to work more efficiently by stimulating the circulation, but can also help to relieve tension (which puts undue stress on the system and restricts the blood flow). For example:

* Lavender is a heart sedative and can help to reduce palpitations and lower blood pressure
* Lemon is a tonic to the circulation and can help to liquefy the blood
* Neroli can aid a poor circulation due to its depurative effect (blood cleaning).

The Lymphatic System

The lymphatic system has three main functions:

* **Drainage of excess fluid from the body cells and tissues**   extra cellular fluid from the tissue is absorbed into the lymphatic vessels and is carried away to the lymph nodes to be cleansed before entering the bloodstream via the subclavian veins.

* **Fighting infection**   the lymph nodes manufacture lymphocytes and generate antibodies, which help to ingest and neutralise invading bacteria. The lymph nodes act as filtering stations and are densely packed with the lymphocytes, which ingest foreign bodies as the lymph (colourless fluid containing white blood cells) passes through the nodes.

✳ **Absorption and distribution of fat-soluble nutrients** upon reaching the small intestine, the products of fat digestion pass into the lymphatic system via intestinal lymphatic vessels called the lacteals.

Aromatherapy places particular importance upon the lymphatic system in that it helps to facilitate several actions:

✳ stimulates immunity

✳ encourages the flow of lymph from the tissues and into the circulatory system

✳ prevents oedema

✳ reduces the viscosity of blood

✳ reduces generalised swelling in the tissues

✳ stimulates the absorption of waste material from the tissues.

Aromatherapy can help the lymphatic system in the following ways:

✳ Diuretic essential oils help to accelerate lymph and tissue fluid circulation, e.g. Fennel, Lemon, Juniper and Geranium.

✳ Essential oils help stimulate the circulatory system, e.g. Black Pepper, Rosemary and Ginger.

✳ Essential oils can help to increase the production of white blood cells to stimulate immunity, e.g. Bergamot, Lavender, Lemon, Chamomile, Rosemary and Thyme.

✳ All essential oils are antiseptic and bactericidal to some extent, but Chamomile, Lavender, Lemon, Clove, Sandalwood and Teatree are probably the most effective in relation to these properties.

The Endocrine System

The endocrine system is a highly sophisticated system of communication and co-ordination, which governs many body processes.

The endocrine glands that make up the system each secrete chemicals (hormones) into the bloodstream. These chemicals can influence parts of the body that are often quite distant from the point of secretion. The main endocrine glands include the following:

✳ pituitary gland

✳ thyroid gland

✳ parathyroid glands

✳ adrenal glands

✳ the islets of langerhans

✳ ovaries

✳ testes.

There are many similarities between an essential oil and a hormone:

✳ both contain chemical compounds

✳ both are transported by the bloodstream

✳ both can help to regulate body processes

* both affect our physical and psychological well-being

* both can have a direct or an indirect effect on the body.

Essential oils appear to act on the endocrine system and on various body functions regulated by the endocrine system, in two ways:

* directly

* indirectly.

Direct effect

Certain essential oils contain plant hormones or *phytohormones*. They can act on the body in the same way as a hormone, in that they directly affect a target organ or tissue. For example, the essential oil of Fennel contains a form of oestrogen in its structure and therefore can be effective for female problems such as pre-menstrual syndrome and the menopause; Rose and Jasmine have a direct effect on the reproductive system and have been used to help stimulate contraction of the uterus in labour, as well as helping with female reproductive problems.

Indirect effect

Essential oils can influence the hormone secretion of the various glands. They act as triggers, stimulating the production of a hormone or a balancing agent, which may either help to raise or reduce the amount of a hormone that is being produced, thereby restoring the endocrine system to a more balanced state. For example, Geranium helps to stimulate the adrenal cortex, which will indirectly influence the secretion of the corticoid hormones: Clary Sage, Lavender and Ylang Ylang all help to lower blood pressure.

The Nervous System

The nervous system is the main communication system for the body and works intimately with the endocrine system to regulate body processes. It has two main divisions:

* the *central nervous system*, which is the control centre and consists of a two-way communication system of the brain and the spinal cord

* the *peripheral* system, consisting of nerves that carry messages to and from the central nervous system.

The central nervous system

The functional unit of the nervous system is a neurone or nerve, and there are two main types of nerve impulses:

* sensory nerves, which receive stimuli from sensory organs and receptors, and transmit the impulses to the spinal cord and brain

* motor nerves, which conduct nerve impulses away from the central nervous system towards muscles and glands, to stimulate them into action.

> ## Key Note
>
> In aromatherapy massage, the sensory stimulus of touch and pressure will be received by the sensory receptors in the skin, and smell will be received by the olfactory receptor cells in the top of the nasal cavity.
>
> Sensory impulses are important for the success of aromatherapy treatment as they will convey both the aroma and the touch associated with massage, along the nerve pathways up the central nervous system to the brain, where they will be perceived by the limbic system.

The most important areas of the brain for aromatherapy are therefore:

* **the olfactory bulb**   in the cerebral cortex, perceives the aroma
* **the limbic system**   known as the 'smell brain', related to emotions and memory
* **the hypothalamus**   regulates other body functions through its control of the endocrine system and autonomic nervous system.

> ## Key Note
>
> The hypothalamus is a structure at the base of the brain and is linked with the rest of the brain and the pituitary gland by a complex network of nerve pathways. It serves as an interface between the mind, the nervous system and endocrine systems.
>
> It controls hunger, thirst, temperature, sexual response and is also closely involved with our emotions and sleep patterns.

The Peripheral Nervous System

The peripheral nervous system is made up of the parts of the nervous system outside the brain and spinal cord. It comprises:

* 31 pairs of spinal nerves
* 12 pairs of cranial nerves
* the autonomic nervous system

The 31 pairs of spinal nerves pass out of the spinal cord. Each has two thin branches that link it with the autonomic nervous system. Spinal nerves receive sensory impulses from the body and transmit motor signals to specific regions of the body. By stimulating the spinal nerves through aromatherapy massage, communication can be made with many of the organs of the body (respiratory, digestive, sensory, urinary and reproductive) and any blockages and weaknesses in the nerve pathways can be assisted to clear.

Aromatherapy can help the nervous system by:

* reducing nervous tension and helping stress-related conditions
* inducing relaxation
* stimulating the nerves to clear congestion in the nerves and thereby improve the functioning of related organs and tissues.

Examples of essential oils that have an affinity for the nervous system include the following:

* Bergamot, Chamomile, Jasmine, Lavender, Neroli, Sweet Marjoram and Ylang Ylang are sedatives and have a calming effect on the central nervous system.
* Peppermint, Lemon and Rosemary have a stimulating effect on the nervous system.
* Chamomile, Clary Sage, Juniper, Lavender, Marjoram and Rosemary are nerve tonics and help to strengthen the nervous system.

The Musculo-skeletal System

Aromatherapy can be effective on both the muscular and skeletal system in the following ways:

* Analgesic essential oils such as Lavender, Chamomile, Rosemary and Marjoram can aid the relaxation of tense and painful muscle fibres, tendons and ligaments.
* Rufebacient essential oils such as Rosemary and Black Pepper can assist in increasing the blood supply to the soft tissues, bones and joints, helping to promote flexibility and reduce the risk of injury.
* Anti-inflammatory essential oils such as Chamomile and Lavender can help to reduce inflammation around joints.
* Detoxifying essential oils such as Lemon and Juniper can assist in eliminating waste products such as lactic acid and uric acid from the tissues.

Key Note

In cases where an area may be too painful to massage, it may be preferable to use a compress to help reduce inflammation, swelling and pain.

Task

Complete the following table to illustrate which essential oils may be effective for the following systems.

Type of	Essential oils that may be effective on the system
Skin	
Respiratory	
Blood Circulation	
Lymphatic	
Endocrine	
Nervous	
Musculo-skeletal	

✳ Table 5: Essential oils and systems of the body ✳

Self-assessment Questions

1. Explain briefly the two main ways in which essential oils are absorbed into the bloodstream for therapeutic effect.

----

2. List the principal parts of the olfactory system.

----

3. Briefly explain the process of olfaction.

----

4. How can a smell stimulate an emotional response within the brain?

----

5. State five similarities between essential oils and hormones.

CHAPTER 7

The Aromatherapy Consultation

A consultation is a very important part of the whole aromatherapy treatment, and should be holistic in its approach. The initial consultation allows the aromatherapist to determine as far as possible the client's needs and will establish whether treatment is appropriate or whether referral to another professional should be the next course of action.

From the information elicited from the consultation, the aromatherapist may then select and blend oils based upon the client's physical and emotional condition, and plan a treatment to suit their needs.

* A competent aromatherapist will develop good communication and client-handling skills, in order to elicit as much information as possible, while at the same time building a good rapport and level of trust with a client.

Objectives

By the end of this chapter you will be able to relate the following knowledge to your work as an aromatherapist:

* relevant factors to be discussed during an aromatherapy consultation to identify clients' needs
* how to keep full and accurate records
* professional etiquette in handling referral data
* guidelines on detailing case studies.

The Purpose of a Consultation

A consultation is the first line of communication between the client and the aromatherapist, and best results are gained through co-operation and good communication between both parties. The purpose of an aromatherapy consultation is to enable the aromatherapist to:

* establish whether the client is suitable for treatment or whether a medical referral is required
* establish the need for any special care, which may involve an adaptation of treatment and oils used
* develop a good rapport with the client

✳ explain what aromatherapy is, along with its benefits

✳ identify the objectives of the treatment

✳ agree a treatment plan with the client to suit their needs

✳ answer the client's questions and allay any fears regarding the nature of the treatment.

The aromatherapy treatment should always commence with a consultation. The aromatherapist will be aware of the client's characteristics and body language from the moment the client walks in; everything will contribute to the overall picture of the client.

A skilled aromatherapist will also be an accomplished listener. S/he will listen carefully to what the client says and empathise with their problems, while also helping them to accept responsibility for their problems, and to accept help from the aromatherapist.

Aromatherapists as professionals must do their utmost to ascertain the nature of any ailment or condition prior to treatment. If any doubt exists about the health of the client and their suitability for treatment, they should be referred to their medical practitioner.

Key Note

If a consultation has been undertaken and a specific medical condition arises, it should be explained to the client why aromatherapy may not be carried out without a doctor's referral.

If the client gives permission, a letter may be sent to the client's GP asking for further information regarding the client's condition, and whether aromatherapy treatment may progress.

The client may wish to take the letter to their GP directly or may wish for the aromatherapist to communicate directly with the doctor by post.

A record of all communication should be made on the consultation noting the date the letter was sent and the date it was received.

NO treatment should be carried out until medical approval has been granted.

If the GP gives approval, it is professional etiquette to keep him/her informed of the progress of the client, along with any results arising from the treatment given.

The information elicited from the consultation will form the basis upon which the aromatherapist makes a selection of appropriate oils to use for treatment. It is essential, therefore, that the client is prepared to disclose any relevant information regarding their health and condition, to enable the aromatherapist to choose suitable oils and avoid those that may be contra-indicated.

Although the initial consultation is generally the most important one for establishing the main factors relating to the client, it is important to remember that consultations are ongoing. Each treatment should be planned individually on each treatment occasion, to ensure that all client details that may affect the treatment are up to date.

Confidentiality

It is very important that records of all consultations are kept confidentially. This should be explained to clients in order to reassure them. Maintaining client confidentiality will show a high degree of professionalism and will prevent embarrassment and loss of client loyalty.

During a consultation, the aromatherapist will need to ask the client personal questions. When asking questions of a personal nature, it is important for the aromatherapist to maintain a polite, sensitive and professional manner and stress that the information is necessary to help establish how you can help them.

When carrying out a consultation, it is important to seat yourselves in a comfortable area, preferably out of earshot of others, and to maintain eye contact throughout. Try to turn the questions into more of a chat rather than sounding as if you are merely completing a form, as this will personalise the treatment and relax the client. If you ask open questions, you will generally find that clients are more co-operative with their responses.

Key Note

Whilst the aromatherapist should always have the client's best interests at heart, it is important to remain positive about the treatment and not to become personally involved with the client's problems.

Aromatherapists must remain professionally detached from the client's problems at all times, otherwise they may become unable to help them.

The Consultation Form

Consultation forms are used to record information regarding the client's health, both past and present, and will highlight the client's present condition in order to establish the basis upon which the treatment will be formed. See pages 135–138 for a sample consultation form.

The main factors to be considered during the consultation include:

Medical history

It is important to know the client's medical history, as certain conditions may contra-indicate or restrict aromatherapy treatment, and a GP referral may be needed prior to the commencement of treatment.

Current medical treatment

If the client is under GP or hospital care, a GP referral will be necessary in order to establish the nature of the treatment and how it might affect the proposed aromatherapy treatment.

Medication

It is necessary to ascertain the type of allopathic medicine prescribed. GP referral may be necessary, as certain medications are incompatible with aromatherapy and may cause unpleasant side effects.

General health

It is important that the client's general health and well-being are discussed during the consultation. This may involve their general immunity, energy levels, stress levels and sleep patterns, which will all contribute to the overall picture of the client.

Emotional state

As our emotions can have a profound effect on the way we feel, it is important to establish the client's emotional state prior to treatments as this may affect the selection of oils chosen. For example, they may wish to feel uplifted or calmed and relaxed.

Lifestyle

A client's lifestyle will play an important part in their general well-being. Information regarding the client's job and home circumstances will often reflect the type of lifestyle they lead. Exercise undertaken is included under the heading of general lifestyle; if the client undertakes no exercise, it could lead to fluid retention, a reduction in the efficiency of the lymphatic system and poor energy levels.

Diet and nutrition

It is important to have information regarding a typical daily diet of the client (including fluid levels), to ensure that they are eating the correct amount of nutrients for correct body functioning. Malnutrition can put stress onto the body and lead to increased stress levels and irritability.

Alcohol consumption and smoking levels are important factors to know about, as these will also affect the health of the client.

Hobbies and relaxation

It is important to discuss whether a client has time for a hobby and relaxation. By having an interest in a hobby, a client is able to relax and unwind, which gives the mind and body a chance to escape everyday stresses and to recuperate.

Record Keeping

It is very important to ensure that a full consultation is undertaken with each client and that a record of each treatment is kept. All records should be kept confidentially and be accurate and up to date.
The treatment record should include the following information:

* results from last treatment (if applicable)

* proposed treatment plan (should take account of length of treatment, areas for treatment, number of treatments and the availability of the client)

* treatment objective

* essential oils blended and reasons for use

* dilution of essential oils used

* after care given

* home care advice given (including blend of oils given to the client for home use)

* outcome of treatment with regard to effectiveness

* recommendations for future treatments.

See page 139 for a sample treatment sheet.

Case Study

Sarah Hobson

Introduction

Sarah is an active 31-year-old Test Manager who enjoys playing softball and volleyball in the summer as well as going hiking. She tries to go to the gym at least twice a week (time and work permitting). Sarah has problems with her back and struggles to get comfortable at night, therefore her sleep patterns are irregular.

Conclusion

During the first session, Sarah was nervous about being touched and protective of her back, initially wriggling about when I touched her. Once she became accustomed to my touch, she relaxed and enjoyed the massages. The treatments had a positive effect and she left my home glowing and relaxed. Sarah decided that aromatherapy massage was definitely her favourite form of treatment.

AROMATHERAPY CONSULTATION FORM

Client Note
The following information is required for your safety and to benefit your health. Whilst essential oils and massage are totally safe when administered professionally by an aromatherapist, there are certain contra-indications that require special attention.

The following details will be treated in the strictest of confidence. It may, however, be necessary for you to consult your GP before any aromatherapy treatment can be given.

Date of initial consultation: 15 January 2003   Client ref. no.: SH10

GENERAL
Name: SARAH HOBSON
Address: 63 AVENUE ROAD, HAMPSHIRE

Telephone Number – Daytime: 80428260   Evening:
Date of Birth: 31 July 1964   Occupation: TEST MANAGER

MEDICAL
Name of Doctor: DR ORDON   Surgery: ST MARKS
Address: LITTLETON LANE   Tel No.: 80489671
          SOUTHWICK

Medical Details

Do you have or have you ever suffered with any of the following:

Circulatory disorder? N
Heart condition? N
High or low Blood Pressure? Y HIGH – MONITORED – STABLE NOW.
Thrombosis? N
Varicose Veins? N
Epilepsy? N
Diabetes? N
Dysfunction of the Nervous System? N
Recent haemorrhage or swelling? N
Recent operation/fracture/sprain? N
Abdominal complaint? IBS
Skin disorder? N
A potentially fatal or terminal condition (e.g. cancer)? N

Female clients

Is it possible that you may be pregnant? N
If pregnant, how many months (any history of miscarriage)? N/A
Are you currently menstruating? N
Number of pregnancies (with dates) –

Are you currently under GP/hospital care?
NO

Current medical treatment
NO

Current medication (list dosages)
NO

GP Referral Required?	Yes ( )		No (u)
Clearance form sent	Yes ( )	No ( )	Date:
Clearance form received	Yes ( )	No ( )	Date:

GENERAL HEALTH

Is your general immunity/health (GOOD)/ AVERAGE / POOR ?

Would you say your energy levels are HIGH /(AVERAGE)/ LOW ?

Would you consider your stress levels to be HIGH /(AVERAGE)/ LOW ?

Sleep patterns? LIGHT SLEEPER – DIFFICULTY GETTING COMFORTABLE

HEALTH RELATED PROBLEMS

Do you suffer with any of the following:

Skin Complaints i.e.
Allergies / Dermatitis / Eczema / Psoriasis / Other?

INTOLERANCE – ONIONS

Problems with Circulation, Muscles, Nerves and Joints i.e.
Arthritis / Muscular aches and pains / Chilblains / Oedema / Rheumatism / Sciatica / Other?

DISLOCATED RIGHT SHOULDER – MARCH 2002

Respiratory problems i.e.
Asthma / Breathing difficulties / Bronchitis / Throat infections, / Sinusitis / Colds / Flu / Other?

SEASONAL

Digestive problems i.e.
Constipation / Indigestion / Colitis / Candida / Other?

IBS

Urinary problems i.e.
Cystitis / Thrush / Fluid Retention / Other?

NO

Nervous/Stress-related problems i.e.
Anxiety / Depression / Headaches / Migraine / Insomnia / Nervous tension / Other?

NO

Female Clients
Pre-menstrual Tension / Menopausal problems / Problems with periods?

PAIN – LIKE CONTRACTIONS
WEEPY – MORNING OF THE FIRST DAY

Is there any other problem that has not been mentioned that you would like help with as part of this treatment?

NO

Summary of client's main presenting problem/s

LIFESTYLE
Typical daily diet:

CEREAL / BAGEL & HONEY
FRUIT – APPLE / BANANA
SALAD & SOUP / JACKET POTATO / SANDWICH
FRUIT
CEREAL / BAGEL
1/2–1 PINT OF MILK

Number of glasses of water consumed daily: 7

Number of cups of tea/coffee per day: 3–4

Vitamins/minerals taken: COD LIVER OIL CAPSULES
    SEA KELP
    VITAMIN C

Typical weekly alcohol consumption   Do you smoke? If so how many daily?
10–15 UNITS   YES   5

Type of exercise undertaken (and how frequently) TWICE WEEKLY
GYM – AEROBIKE – CARDIOVASCULAR
WALKING

Do you have any hobbies? Do you relax regularly, if so how? VOLLEYBALL, SOFTBALL
                |
HIKING   HOT BATH (SOAK)

Have you tried aromatherapy or any other complementary therapies before?
(state when and what the results were)   LAVENDAR SLEEP SACK

Are you currently having any complementary treatment? (give details)   PHYSIOTHERAPY

CLIENT DECLARATION

I declare that the information I have given is correct and as far as I am aware I can undertake treatment with this establishment without any adverse effects. I have been fully informed about contra-indications and I am therefore willing to proceed with the treatment.

Client's Signature: *Sarah Adson*   **Date:** 15/1/03

Therapist's Signature: *Joanne*

Notes

OVER-PRODUCTION OF STOMACH ACID – MEDICATION 1 MONTH

✳ **Figure 21: A sample consultation form** ✳

AROMATHERAPY TREATMENT RECORD

CLIENT REFERENCE NUMBER: _____

Date	Feedback from last treatment	Treatment needs/ objectives	Treatment plan (state method of application)	Essential oils used (state no. of drops)	Reasons for choice	Dilution rate	Carrier oils/ other vehicle used (state mls used)	Parts of body treated	Results	Home care advice given
15/1/03		General well-being	Massage	Jasmine = 2 Orange = 2 Frankincense = 1	anti-inflammatory IBS sedative	1%	Sweet Almond 20 ml	A; B; C; D; E	Client was thirsty	ALL
				Ylang Ylang = 1	skin care	1%	Jojoba 5 ml	F; G		
		Menstrual pain	Oil	Jasmine = 3 Geranium = 1 Grapefruit = 3	menstrual pain hormone balancer fluid retention	+2%	Sweet Almond 10 ml	E		Avoid contact with eyes
11/2/03	Relaxed Slept well Energised the following day	Destress	Massage	Bergamot = 2 Patchouli = 2 Chamomile = 2 Geranium = 1	stress stress calming skin care	<2% 1%	Sweet Almond 20 ml Jojoba 5 ml	A; B; C; D; E F; G	Relaxed and floaty	ALL
		Relaxing Promote sleep	Bubble-bath (for use at night)	Orange = 4 Marjoram = 5 Ylang Ylang = 6	IBS; sleep muscle relaxant insomnia	+2%	Base Bubble-bath 50 ml Wheatgerm 10 drops	A; B; C; D; E F; G		Avoid contact with eyes B
15/2/03	Relaxed and happy	Relaxing	Massage	Neroli = 3 Bergamot = 2 Sandalwood = 1 Jasmine = 1	stress relief calming stress sedative skin care	<2% 1%	Sweet Almond 20 ml Jojoba 5 ml	A; B; C; D; E F; G	Relaxed	ALL

✳ **Figure 22: A sample treatment sheet** ✳

139

> **Key Note**
>
> It is very important to review the client's treatment plan at regular intervals, along with the oils used. Care should be taken to avoid using the same blend of oils for an extended period of time, to avoid the client's building up sensitivity to any oil or oils used. Due to the diversity of properties of essential oils, there will always be a suitable alternative, preventing the need to use the same oils each time.

> **Task**
>
> Practise carrying out detailed consultations on clients in preparation for an aromatherapy treatment. These may form part of your portfolio of evidence, to compile aromatherapy case studies.
>
> Each consultation you carry out should include the following information in relation to the client:
>
> * personal details
> * medical history
> * current medical treatment
> * medication
> * emotional state
> * lifestyle and diet
> * reasons for treatment

Guidelines for Case Studies

A client case study is a record of a series of treatments that have been undertaken on a client and have been evaluated for their effectiveness.

A complete case study will generally consist of the following parts:

* A general introduction to the client to include their background information such as present condition, lifestyle and emotional state, along with the main treatment objectives.

* A completed consultation form, which is detailed and elicits their physical and emotional state, and all other relevant factors.

* A record of all treatments undertaken and an evaluation of their effectiveness.

* Summary and conclusion after a course of treatments has been given. You may ask the client to complete a feedback sheet or give a testimonial.

Key Note

Remember that client case studies contain confidential information, therefore it is important to obtain the client's written permission that they do not object to details being kept in your portfolio.

Self-assessment Questions

1. *State two important reasons for undertaking a consultation prior to aromatherapy treatment.*

----

2. *Why is it important to keep full and accurate records on aromatherapy treatments given for each client?*

----

3. *State ten factors that should be discussed with a client during a consultation for aromatherapy.*

----

4. Explain the procedure and etiquette for dealing with referral data for aromatherapy treatments.

CHAPTER 8

Blending in Aromatherapy

> *The art of blending essential oils is one of the most creative parts of an aromatherapy practice. When essential oils are blended together, their molecules combine to form a synergy so that the combination of essential oils or the 'whole' becomes more than the sum of its individual parts.*
>
> *The art of true aromatherapy therefore lies in selecting and blending oils to create synergistic blends.*

✳ A competent aromatherapist will have a thorough knowledge of the therapeutic properties of essential oils, and will be able to select and blend oils individually for each client.

Objectives

By the end of this chapter you will be able to relate the following knowledge to your work carried out as an aromatherapist:

✳ the principles of synergy and blending

✳ factors to be considered when blending essential oils

✳ quantities and proportions when blending essential oils

✳ the therapeutic properties and uses of carrier oils.

Synergy

When two or more oils are blended together, the chemistry of the oils combines with one another to create an entirely new substance whose properties as a whole add up to more than the sum of its individual parts. By blending together mutually enhancing oils, the interaction of the various molecular components creates a synergistic blend, which is more powerful than using an individual oil on its own.

Furthermore, the principle of synergy allows the therapist to be accurate in providing treatments by taking into account all factors relating to the client, both physical and psychological, and creating a blend to suit their individual needs and condition.

The principle of synergy was strongly advocated by Marguerite Maury when she introduced the idea of the 'individual prescription' in the 1950s.

> ## Key Note
>
> The principle of synergy is context-dependent, which means that a successful synergistic blend created for one client may be wholly inappropriate for another client. A synergistic blend therefore treats the person in a *holistic* way by taking account of all aspects of that person, rather than treating them for an isolated condition.

Blending

Blending essential oils is an individual skill and there are many ways in which it can be undertaken.

Firstly, in order to be able to blend essential oils successfully, you will need to study the therapeutic properties of the oils to understand their effects and their individual characters (see Chapter 4), as well as having personal experience of using the oils.

Personal experimentation is the only way to learn, as essential oils possess an array of therapeutic possibilities that can be blended into endless combinations.

There are many factors to consider when blending essential oils:

Proportions

When blending it is important to remember that essential oils are very powerful and concentrated substances; it is often the minute proportions of an essential oil that can effect the healing process.

For aromatherapy massage, a dilution of 2 per cent of essential oil to carrier oil is usually recommended.

An easy way of remembering the number of essential oil drops to carrier oil is to divide the mls of carrier oil you are using by two. For example, if you are using 30 ml of carrier oil, you could add *up to* 15 drops of essential oil to make your blend.

> ## Key Note
>
> In aromatherapy, it does not always follow that the more you use, the better the effect will be; the reverse is often the case. Some aromatherapists may use more or less than a 2 per cent dilution to achieve the desired effects, but the most important overriding factor is that the proportions used are sensible and are within safety guidelines to avoid undesired effects.

It is also important to consider the odour intensity of the oils being used as some may predominate so will need to be used in small amounts to create a balanced blend.

Client type

The type of client to be treated will always influence the essential oils blended. For children and pregnant women it is recommended that a 1 per cent dilution is used and there are several essential oils that should not be used (see Chapter 2).

Area being treated

Unless the client has a very sensitive skin, it is usual to use a 2 per cent dilution of essential oils for therapeutic body work. However, when working on sensitive areas such as the face, a 1 per cent dilution is recommended.

Do remember also to consider your choice of oils when working on the face; some may be too stimulating, for example Marjoram and Black Pepper.

Compatibility

Certain essential oils are mutually enhancing and will blend well together, whereas some have an inhibiting effect on each other. Personal experimentation is the only way of finding which oils blend well together, but it is worth considering that botanical families of oils blend well with each other; for example, members of the herb family (Lavender, Marjoram, Rosemary) blend well with citrus (Lemon, Orange, Bergamot) and flowers (Rose, Ylang Ylang, Jasmine).

Notes

The classification of essential oils into notes originates from the perfumery industry, where it is said that a well-balanced perfume contains a top, middle and base note. This principle is not used in quite the same way for aromatherapy as for perfumery, although it may be useful to take account of notes to ensure that the blend you create is well-balanced from an aesthetic point of view.

* Top notes are the fastest acting essences and give the first impression in a blend as they are highly volatile.
* Middle notes are less volatile and usually form the heart of the blend.
* Base notes are the least volatile and act as blend fixatives to make the aroma last longer.

Aesthetics

Although we are principally blending essential oils for therapeutic reasons, it is a good idea to take into account the aesthetics of the aroma to ensure you create a balanced blend. Smell is a very powerful sense and if the aroma of the blend is not pleasing to the client, the overall objectives may not be met as the client might not be able to relax and enjoy the full benefits of the treatment.

It is therefore very important to consider the odour intensity of the oils you intend to blend, as some oils are highly odiferous and may need to be toned down with other, less powerful and more balancing oils.

Client preference

The client's choice of aroma is often very personal, as blends react with the individual chemistry of a person's skin to create an entirely unique aroma.

> ## Key Note
>
> It is important to remember that odours are multifaceted and a single odiferous material may be composed of many different overtones and undertones. It is for this reason that some clients may perceive a particular aroma quite differently from others.
>
> Even the mood of the client can affect the way in which the aroma of a blend of essential oils is perceived.

Cost

It is important to blend only as much as you need for an individual treatment to ensure cost-effectiveness. Treatment is not always improved by adding several essential oils, and it is wasteful to use several oils for the sake of blending if fewer oils would fit the overall purpose.

By using a maximum of three or four essential oils to a blend, you will keep in touch with the individual aroma and qualities of the oils as you start to create synergistic blends.

Treatment objective and individual needs of client

As you are creating a synergistic blend it is essential to take account of the client's predominant problems (both physical and emotional) along with an overall treatment objective, to ensure the client's needs are being met. For example, does the client need general relaxation physically but an uplift emotionally?

Client's skin type

The client's skin type may often influence your choice of essential oils. For example, if your client suffers from skin problems, the dilution and type of oils must be carefully selected to avoid adverse skin reactions.

Variations in blending

There are many accepted variations in blending techniques, which will often be unique to the person creating the blend. A good analogy is to imagine following a recipe book, while at the same time adding in one's own interpretation or ingredients to make it unique.

Some aromatherapists use dowsing or crystals to assist them in their selection of oils for a client, while others use the Eastern principle of yin (being calming and relaxing) and yang (being stimulating). Certain aromatherapists are guided by their intuition, based upon their knowledge of the therapeutic effects and characteristics of each oil.

When blending, your nose is generally the best guide, combined with personal experimentation and experience. Whichever method of blending is used, these important factors must be considered:

* Is the blend of oils created acceptable to the client?

* Does the blend meet with the treatment objective?

* Has the blend been created synergistically, taking into account all relevant factors relating to the client?

* Are the proportions used within safe limits?

Properties and Uses of Carrier Oils

In order to aid their absorption into the bloodstream, essential oils are carried by base or vegetable carrier oils. Carrier oils are commonly referred to as fixed oils, as they act as blending or stabilising agents for the essential oils. In addition, they have therapeutic benefits of their own, which can enhance the effectiveness of the blend.

Carrier oils used in aromatherapy should preferably be unrefined or cold pressed. The refining process of vegetable oils is undesirable in the practice of aromatherapy, as the oils are produced by intense heat, which has a destructive effect on the aroma, colour and its natural constituents (i.e. vitamins, minerals and enzymes).

Unrefined oils are superior in comparison as they retain their natural constituents, which are therapeutically beneficial for the skin and the body's systems. The main method used for extracting vegetable carrier oils is cold or warm pressing: the oil seed, nut or kernel is heated at a low temperature to help release the oil, and is then put through a cold press.

The choice of carrier oil used in a blend will be primarily dependent on the client's skin type and the therapeutic objectives of the treatment.

In aromatherapy, it is best to use carrier oils with little or no odour to allow the essential oils to work effectively.

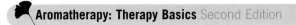
Common Carrier Oils used in Aromatherapy

Apricot kernel

> ### Key Note
>
> Apricot kernel is generally too expensive to use on its own so it may be blended with other less expensive carriers such as grapeseed and sweet almond. It is very effective for therapeutic massage and is light enough for facial massage.

Botanical name: *Prunus armenica*
Source: extracted from the seed kernel of the fruit
Colour: pale yellow
Contains: vitamins and minerals, notably vitamin A
Therapeutic properties: very easily absorbed, nourishing and soothing
Skin types suitable for: all skin types, especially dry, sensitive, mature and inflamed

Avocado

> ### Key Note
>
> As this oil is fairly viscous, highly odorous and relatively expensive, use as a 10 per cent addition to another lighter carrier.

Botanical name: *Persea americana*
Source: cold pressed from the flesh of the avocado fruit
Colour: dark green
Therapeutic properties: soothing, relives itching, highly penetrative. Contains: protein, lecithin, essential fatty acids, vitamins A, B and D
Skin types suitable for: all skin types, especially dry, dehydrated and sensitive

Calendula (Pot Marigold)

> ## Key Note
>
> The oil is especially gentle and soothing for use with children, babies and those with sensitive skin.

Botanical name: *Calendula officinalis*
Source: macerated from the flowers
Colour: orange-yellow
Therapeutic properties: anti-inflammatory, astringent, softening and soothing on the skin, healing
Skin types suitable for: all skin types, especially dry and sensitive

Evening primrose

> ## Key Note
>
> This oil is reputed to be effective for menopausal problems and pre-menstrual syndrome. It is a very expensive oil so use as a 10 per cent dilution to other carrier oils; alternatively, buy in capsule form and add one or two capsules to the blend.

Botanical name: *Oenothera biennis*
Source: extracted from the seeds
Colour: pale yellow
Therapeutic properties: soothing and nourishing, reputed to help accelerate healing in the body. Contains polyunsaturated fatty acids and is rich in linoleic acid
Skin types suitable for: all skin types, especially dry

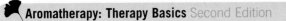
Grapeseed

> ## Key Note
>
> This oil has a very light texture and is effective for general massage purposes. It can therefore be used on its own as a carrier, but is more commonly used as the main basic oil and other oils with more nutrients are added to it.

Botanical name: *Vitis vinifera*
Source: heat extracted from the grape pips of the fruit
Colour: pale green
Therapeutic properties: gentle emollient. Contains linoleic acid, protein and a small proportion of vitamin E. Free from cholesterol
Skin types suitable for: all skin types

Hazelnut

> ## Key Note
>
> This oil is quickly absorbed for massage purposes and can be used as a 100 per cent carrier, although it does tend to be expensive.

Botanical name: *Corylus avellana*
Source: extracted from hazelnuts
Colour: yellow
Therapeutic properties: has a slightly astringent effect on the skin and is stimulating to the circulation. Good penetrative qualities. Contains oleic acid (monosaturated fatty acid) and linoleic acid (polyunsaturated fatty acid). Contains vitamin E
Skin types suitable for: all skin types, especially oily or combination skins

Jojoba

Key Note

Key Note

This oil is light and fine in texture and is very effective for facial and body massage. As it is rich and expensive, it may be added to other carriers or used on its own.

Botanical name: *Simmondsia chinensis*
Source: extracted from the bean of the plant
Colour: yellow (liquid wax)
Therapeutic properties: anti-inflammatory, highly penetrative. Its chemical structure resembles sebum and contains a waxy substance that mimics collagen. Rich in vitamin E, protein and minerals. Natural moisturiser
Skin types suitable for: all skin types including oily, combination, acne skins and inflamed skins

Macadamia nut

Key Note

This oil has become a very popular carrier in aromatherapy due to its nutritive properties.

Botanical name: *Macadamia integrifolia* and *Macadamia ternifolia*
Source: warm pressed from the plant
Colour: peach colour
Therapeutic properties: highly emollient, rich and nutritive. Contains essential fatty acids found in sebum
Skin types suitable for: all skin types, especially for dry and ageing skins

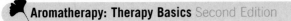

Olive oil

> ### Key Note
>
> **This oil is very heavy and viscous, and tends to have a strong odour.**

Botanical name: *Olea Europaea*
Source: extracted from hard, unripe olives
Colour: yellow-green
Therapeutic properties: rich and nutritive, contains a good source of vitamin E. Very soothing
Skin types suitable for: dehydrated skins and inflamed skin

Peach kernel

> ### Key Note
>
> **This oil has a regenerative and tonic effect on the skin.**

Botanical name: *Prunus persica*
Source: extracted from the kernel
Colour: pale green
Therapeutic properties: emollient, helps increase skin suppleness and elasticity. Contains vitamins A and E, and some essential fatty acids
Skin types suitable for: all skin types, especially dry and mature

Rosehip

Key Note

Rosehip has a rich texture and therefore should be diluted with another carrier oil (50/50). It is an excellent oil to use on the scar following surgery as it helps to aid a speedy recovery.

Botanical name: *Rosa cannina*
Source: extracted from the seeds of the rosehip
Colour: rose
Therapeutic properties: has the same polyunsaturated fatty acids as human skin (linoleic acid); regenerating and healing
Skin types suitable for: scar tissue, stretch marks, dehydrated skins

Safflower

Key Note

This oil is very economical to use as a carrier as it is inexpensive and light.

Botanical name: *Carthamux tinctorius*
Source: warm pressed from the seeds
Colour: yellow
Therapeutic properties: nutritive, as rich in essential fatty acids and vitamin E
Skin types suitable for: all skin types

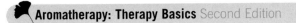

St Johns wort

> **Key Note**
>
> This oil is specially effective on healing wounds and for soothing inflammation.

Botanical name: *Hypericum perforatum*
Source: macerated from the flowers and leaves
Colour: mauvey-red-brown
Therapeutic properties: anti-inflammatory, astringent, soothing and healing to the skin
Skin types suitable for: all skin types, especially dry and sensitive

Sunflower

> **Key Note**
>
> This oil is very fine and light and is a relatively neutral oil, making it effective for general purposes. It is relatively inexpensive.

Botanical name: *Helianthus annus*
Source: warm pressed from the sunflower seeds
Colour: golden yellow
Therapeutic properties: nutritive, contains fatty acids and high levels of vitamin E. Its structure is close to sebum
Skin types suitable for: all skin types, especially dry

Sweet almond

Botanical name: *Prunus amygdalus*
Source: warm pressed from the kernel of the sweet almond tree
Colour: pale yellow
Therapeutic properties: soothing and calming and helps relieve itching. Contains vitamins A, B1, B2, B6, E and is rich in protein. Contains a high proportion of fatty acids
Skin types suitable for: all skin types, especially dry, ageing and inflamed skins

Wheatgerm

Botanical name: *Triticum vulgare*
Source: warm pressed from the germ of the wheat kernel
Colour: orange brown
Therapeutic properties: soothing, nourishing, healing. A natural anti-oxidant. A rich source of vitamin E and protein
Skin types suitable for: all skin types, especially inflamed and ageing

Summary

Key Note

* Carrier oils should be stored in a cold place for up to approximately nine months, after which time they will oxidise.

* As carrier oils are perishable products, it is wise to buy them frequently and in sensible proportions.

How to Blend Oils for Aromatherapy Massage

The equipment needed to mix your essential oils will include the following:

* clear glass or plastic measuring container in ml

* selected essential oils

* selected carrier oils

* selection of dark glass bottles, i.e. 5 ml, 10 ml, 15 ml and 25 ml

* glass rod for stirring

* labels.

Method

* The amount of carrier/s required for the proposed treatment is measured out into the clear glass or plastic container, or directly into a dark glass bottle.

* The number of selected essential oil drops are then added one at a time, remembering to use a 2 per cent dilution for the body and 1 per cent for the face.

* If using a glass or plastic container, it is necessary to stir the mix with a glass rod or other suitable implement such as a spatula. If pouring into a bottle, the lid should be placed on the bottle and the bottle shaken to disperse the essential oils into the carrier.

* If using a bottle, it is important to pour the oil up to the shoulder level of the bottle in order to leave an air gap.

Key Note

Always remember to label the blend if blending into bottles. If reusing the container and bottles, make sure that both are washed thoroughly and disinfected, to remove all trace of the previous blend of oils.

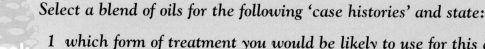

Task

Select a blend of oils for the following 'case histories' and state:

1 which form of treatment you would be likely to use for this client;

2 the choice of essential oils and carrier oil/s used, along with the dilutions; and

3 what home care advice you would offer this client.

* Miss S has cellulite and poor circulation. She also suffers with frequent headaches and has sensitive and dry skin.

* Mr N is an asthmatic with breathing difficulties. Also suffers with eczema and nervous tension. He has oily skin.

* Mrs D suffers extreme tension due to pressure of work, aches and muscular pains in the lumbar region of the back due to bending and lifting at work. Has normal skin, slightly dry.

* Mr J has mild hypertension and occasionally suffers with palpitations. He has just got over the breakdown of his marriage of 20 years and feels very inadequate. Has dry, sensitive skin.

* Miss K suffers with PMT and gets very irritable before a period, which is affecting her relationships at home. She also gets a lot of fluid retention and suffers with migraine. Has normal skin.

* Mrs Y has been taking tranquillisers for over 20 years, which were prescribed originally due to a nervous breakdown, following a bereavement of a close family member. She is very tense and complains of headaches and neck pain. Also has disturbing nightmares.

Self-assessment Questions

1. What is meant by the term 'synergy' in aromatherapy?

----

2. *State five important factors to be taken into account when blending essential oils.*

----

3. *What determines a choice of essential oils for a client in an aromatherapy treatment?*

----

4. *What determines the choice of carrier oil used for a client in aromatherapy?*

----

5. *List the therapeutic properties of the following carrier oils, indicating which skin type/s they may be suitable for:*

   i   Sweet almond

----

ii Grapeseed

----

iii Avocado

----

iv Wheatgerm

----

v Jojoba

CHAPTER 9
Energy-based Concepts in Aromatherapy

> *If energy is not flowing freely in the body, it can result in blockages in the energy pathways, which can lead to imbalances.*
>
> *In order for aromatherapists to understand how emotions can cause energy blocks in the tissues of our body, it is helpful to have an insight into the oriental systems of body circuits, called meridians, and the subtle energy fields of chakras.*
>
> *Essential oils are universal balancers in that they have a range of energetic actions that can help to restore a range of imbalances.*

* A competent aromatherapist needs to have an insight into the energetic concepts of yin and yang, meridians and chakras in order to understand how they relate to physical and emotional balance.

Objectives

By the end of this chapter you will be able to relate the following knowledge in relation to the energetic profiles of essential oils and your work as an aromatherapist:

* the role of yin and yang
* the role of meridians
* the role of chakras.

Yin and Yang

In order to understand imbalance, it is important to explore the oriental concept of yin and yang: the philosophy that forms the foundation of Chinese medicine.

Yin and yang is a way of expressing opposite and complementary states of energy, such as hot and cold, male and female, night and day, winter and summer.

When the yin and yang are balanced within the context of life, health and well-being are experienced; when they are imbalanced ill health can arise.

Everybody, whatever their gender, possesses varying degrees of yin and yang characteristics. The subtle balance is constantly changing, much in the same way as every aspect of the universe changes, such as the cycles of light and the seasons, which are reflective of the constant shift between the polar opposites.

It is important to note that the terms used to describe yin and yang are relative rather than absolute states, therefore there is nothing that is purely yin or purely yang; each contains a part of the other in order to represent wholeness.

Understanding the energetic roles of yin and yang is the key to any therapeutic application such as aromatherapy.

* The primary function of yin is to cool, moisten, relax and promote sleep.

* The primary function of yang is to warm, energise and stimulate.

If a client's yang energy is *deficient* they are likely to feel chilly, tired and unmotivated, and therefore they will be imbalanced towards the yin. In this case, they will benefit from essential oils with a 'yang' (warming, energising) character such as Rosemary or Ginger.

If a client's yang energy is *excessive* they will tend to feel restless, hyperactive and suffer from insomnia, and the imbalance will be towards the yang. In this case they will benefit from essential oils to reduce excess yang, oils that are more yin in character (cooling and relaxing) such as German Chamomile and Melissa.

If a person's yin energy is *deficient* the symptoms are likely to be a feeling of heat, thirst and restlessness. Although similar in character to the symptoms of excess yang, the difference is that the feeling of heat is limited to the hands, feet and chest. Examples of essential oils that help to balance the body's yin energy are Rose and Geranium.

These are examples of excessive or deficient yin and yang states; however, in practice most people are likely to suffer from combinations of yin and yang conditions.

In order to help clients restore balance and overall health, we can use the energetic concepts of yin and yang as a guide; we need to balance the opposing extremes, in other words, the extreme yang part must relax and become more yin and the extreme yin must become more active, or more yang.

The balancing of a client's energy, or yin and yang, can be supported by a choice of particular essential oils that reflect the individual's constitution and character.

Key Note

Due to the relativity of the energetic states of yin and yang, it is significant to note that no essential oil can be categorised as totally 'yin' or totally 'yang'.

Meridians

The human body is like a natural energy source, generating electrical energy within the ionic environment of the cells and tissues. Body meridians contain a colourless free-flowing non-cellular fluid, which conveys electrical energy throughout the body.

The body's circuit of electrical energy is divided into 14 major meridians; there are 12 organic meridians and 2 storage meridians.

Although the meridians are divided in terms of the organs and tissues that they supply, they actually form a single continuous circuit that conveys electromagnetic energy throughout the body.

Having a deeper understanding of meridians can help aromatherapists to recognise that problems in a specific part of the body correspond to problems in specific organs; therefore we can then work on these areas in aromatherapy in order to help address the imbalance.

Key Note

Optimum results will be achieved when aromatherapists can detect which organs and systems are at the root cause of the imbalances, and select the essential oils to help address the deficiency or excess appropriately.

A client's condition, whether excessively yin or yang, will have a direct impact on how the energy flows in the meridians. An excessively cold condition may restrict the flow of energy along a meridian, while too much heat may cause an excess of energy to flow along a meridian.

Body meridians are named according to the internal structures they supply and each of the organic meridians supplies a group of muscles in the body as well as a group of internal tissues.

Six of the organic meridians are called yin meridians. The yin circuit conveys negative electromagnetic energy throughout the body and supplies the yin organs:

* heart
* lungs
* liver

* spleen
* kidney
* pericardium

The yin meridians all have a common purpose in altering, circulating, storing blood and energy (chi) and are deep in the body.

The remaining six organic circuits are called yang meridians. The yang meridians convey positive electromagnetic energy throughout the body and supply the yang organs:

* stomach
* small intestine
* large intestine
* gall bladder

* urinary bladder
* triple warmer (the three zones of energy in the torso)

The yang meridians are closer to the surface and are all part of the digestive system.

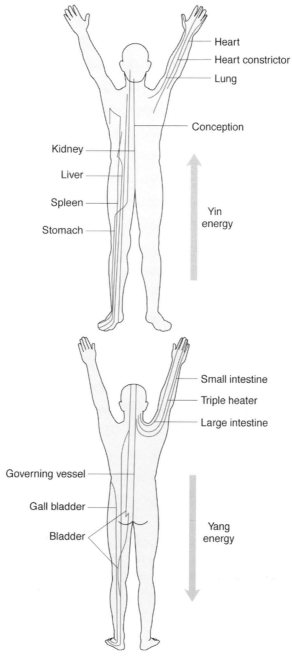

* **Figure 23: *The meridians*** *

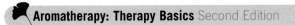

It is important to understand that no organ operates independently within the meridian network. Each yin organ and its meridian works in line with a corresponding organ and meridian. The meridians function in pairs, each one being made up of one yin meridian and one yang meridian. Energy or chi moves from the head towards the feet through the yang meridians on the back of the body and from the feet to the head through the yin meridians on the front.

Heart meridian

The heart meridian begins at the heart and surfaces in the centre of the axilla. The meridian passes down the inside of the arm, crosses the inner point of the elbow fold, and runs through to the tip of the little finger.

Common symptoms of imbalance

Physical

* hot or cold hands and feet
* red complexion
* nervousness
* irritability
* mental or emotional disturbance
* insomnia, disturbed sleep or excessive dreaming

* cardiovascular disorders
* brain or nervous system disorders
* speech problems
* spontaneous sweating
* poor memory of important life events

Emotional

* excessive laughter
* hysteria

* lack of joy
* expressionless appearance

> ## Key Note
> **The heart meridian is the centre of emotional and mental consciousness. It is associated with passion, mental clarity and joy.**

Lung meridian

The lung meridian runs from deep in the body at the lung to surface in the hollow area by the front shoulder. It then passes over the shoulder and down the front of the arm along the biceps muscle. It goes down the arm to the wrist just below the base of the thumb and ends at the thumbnail.

Common symptoms of imbalance

Physical

* asthma
* bronchitis
* congestion in the chest
* coughing
* breathing difficulties
* pneumonia

* excessive mucus
* sore throat
* loss of voice
* deficient or excessive perspiration
* collapsed or hollow chest

Emotional

* chronic or long-term grief, sorrow
* claustrophobia

* compulsive behaviour
* restlessness

> **Key Note**
>
> In Chinese medicine, the lungs are the rulers of energy. How deeply we breathe shapes the energy and gives it its definition.

Liver meridian

The liver meridian begins as a point inside the big toenail, passes over the top of the foot, continues above the inside of the ankle, runs past the inside of the knee and along the inner thigh. It proceeds through the genital region, upward to the sides of the body and then to the ribs just over the liver (for the meridian on the right side of the body) and just over the spleen (on the left side).

Common symptoms of imbalance

Physical

* red face
* pale, drawn face
* headaches (at the top of the head)
* migraines
* dizziness
* pain and swelling in the genitals

* disorders of the eye and vision
* muscle spasms, seizures, convulsions
* pale fingernails, ridges in nails, cracked nails
* pain relating to tendons
* allergies
* easily bruised

* menstrual pain, irregular periods, blood clotting, premenstrual syndrome

* dandruff and hair loss

Emotional

* anger
* frustration

* depression
* lack of will

Key Note

In Chinese medicine, the liver and liver meridian are considered to be the controller of the life force. The liver meridian is associated with expression of the will and with creativity – when life energy is weak it is usually indicative of the liver being troubled.

Spleen meridian

The spleen meridian begins at the inside of the big toe at the nail and then runs along the inside of the foot, it turns upward in front of the ankle bone, then ascends along the inside of the calf to the knee. From there the meridian runs up through the genital region, through the abdomen, proceeds to the spleen itself, and then to the stomach. The meridian continues upward, along the side of the body and chest area to the outside of the breast.

Common symptoms of imbalance

Physical

* digestive problems – dyspepsia, constipation and diarrhoea
* heartburn, acid indigestion
* nausea
* belching and gas
* immune deficiency or disorders
* lymphatic problems (swollen lymph nodes)
* abdominal distension

* appetite imbalance
* hypoglycaemia or diabetes
* heavy, aching body
* knee or thigh problems
* memory problems
* vomiting after eating

Emotional

* excessive worry
* sensitivity

* obsession
* lack of awareness

> ## Key Note
>
> In Chinese medicine, the spleen is regarded as the primary organ of digestion, passing Chi to the small and large intestines. When the spleen is weakened by excessive consumption of sugar and acidic foods, it is unable to pass on sufficient energy to the intestines, which often results in chronic indigestion and constipation

Kidney meridian

The kidney meridian starts at the little toe and crosses under the foot to the inner edge of the instep. It circles the anklebone towards the heel, then rises along the inside of the calf to the inner thigh. At the pubic region it goes internal for a short distance and re-emerges over the abdomen and chest to the clavicle.

Common symptoms of imbalance

Physical

* cold extremities (especially the feet)
* achy or weak bones
* darkness under the eyes
* drowsiness, lack of energy
* diarrhoea
* dizziness on standing
* tinnitus
* oedema
* hearing loss

* low back pain
* irregular menstruation
* pre-menstrual syndrome
* reproductive problems
* soles of feet painful or hot
* urinary incontinence
* sexual problems
* hypertension
* hair loss

Emotional

* fearful, easily frightened
* chronic anxiety

* foolhardiness

> ## Key Note
>
> In Chinese medicine, the kidneys are responsible for strength and constitutional vitality of the body. They control the essential energy within each cell of the body and thereby maintain the health, vitality and function of every organ, system and sense.

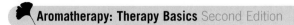

Circulation/Pericardium meridian

The circulation/pericardium meridian starts internally at the surface of the heart and emerges just outside each nipple. It follows around the axilla and travels down the inside of the arm to the wrist, ending at the thumb-side corner of the middle fingernail.

Common symptoms of imbalance

Physical

* stiffness or spasm in the arm and elbow
* distended chest and ribs
* discomfort in chest
* hot palms
* red face

* excessive laughter
* sexual dysfunction
* painful or swollen underarm
* tension in upper chest
* painful, stiff head and neck

Emotional

* timidity
* anxiety
* nervousness

* insensitivity
* rude behaviour

> ## Key Note
>
> **The circulation/pericardium meridian does not correspond directly to an organ.**

Stomach meridian

The stomach meridian starts below the eyes, descends to the sides of the mouth and the jaw, from which a branch rises to the forehead. It continues along the side of the throat to the collarbone and over the chest and abdomen to the pubic area. From there, it passes along the front of the thigh to the outside of the kneecap. Below the kneecap, the meridian divides into two branches, one that ends at the second toe and one that ends at the third toe.

Common symptoms of imbalance

Physical

* abdominal distension (upper)
* abdominal pain
* jaw tension
* knee pain
* lip or mouth sores

* vomiting
* frequent hunger or thirst
* neck or throat swelling
* yawning
* groaning

Emotional

* critical
* lack of understanding
* lack of compassion

* anxiety and nervous tension
* emotionally unstable

Key Note

In Chinese medicine, the stomach and spleen are seen as being connected, one providing energy to the other. As the stomach meridian begins at the mouth, it is said to control the mouth, tongue and oesophagus, thereby controlling the preparation of food for digestion.

Small intestine meridian

The small intestine meridian begins at the outside of the nail on the little finger, trails the back of the hand to the wrist and flows from the outside of the ulna to the elbow. It follows the back of the arm up to the shoulder joint, where it crosses the scapula to the clavicle. From here, the meridian continues up the side of the neck and over the cheek to the ear.

Common symptoms of imbalance

Physical

* abdominal distension (lower)
* arm pain
* shoulder pain and tension
* swollen cheeks

* difficulty in head turning to one side
* sore or stiff elbow joint
* eye soreness or redness
* disorders relating to the small intestine

Emotional

* lack of mental clarity (deficient qi)
* lack of joy (deficient qi)

* over emotional (excess qi)
* hysteria (excess qi)

> ### Key Note
>
> In Chinese medicine, imbalances in the small intestine prevent the smooth transfer of energy from the food to the stomach, resulting in digestive disorders.
>
> In Chinese medicine, the small intestine is seen as linked with the heart, helping to bring clarity of mind.

Large intestine meridian

The large intestine meridian starts at the index finger on the outside of the nail (towards the thumb), runs through the crease between the thumb and the index finger, then passes up the thumb-side edge of the arm to the edge of the shoulder. It then crosses the shoulder and neck to the cheek, touches the upper lip and ends at the nostril.

Common symptoms of imbalance

Physical

* constipation
* diarrhoea
* headache

* shoulder pain
* nasal congestion
* toothache

Emotional

* excessive worry
* grief and sadness

* compulsive attention to detail
* stubbornness

> ### Key Note
>
> In Chinese medicine, the large intestine is recognised as performing the function of elimination in a physical and metaphorical sense. That is, the condition of the large intestine reflects the mind and body's capacity to eliminate those experiences, beliefs and emotions we no longer need in order that we may grow as individuals.
>
> The large intestine is also responsible for sending energy downwards into the body and thus grounding us to the earth.

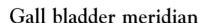

Gall bladder meridian

The first thing to notice about the gall bladder meridian is that it zigzags back and forth over the head and down both sides of the body. It is also one of the longest. The meridian begins at the outside corner of each eye, loops around the ear to the neck, goes back over the head to the forehead above the eyes, then over the head again to the back of the neck. From there it drops down the neck and over the front of each shoulder. It then zigzags down the sides of the body, along the outside of each leg, over the front of the ankles, and ends at the fourth toe.

Common symptoms of imbalance

Physical

* headache (temple) and migraine
* eye and ear pain
* joint stiffness and pain
* tightness and pain in sides of chest
* nausea and vomiting
* yellow colour in eyes
* stiffness in fourth toe
* gall stones

Emotional

* anger and frustration (excess qi)
* depression and lack of will (deficient qi)

Key Note

In Chinese medicine, the gall bladder is seen as an external manifestation of the liver energy, therefore liver symptoms become more pronounced when the gall bladder is imbalanced.

The Chinese say that when the gall bladder is balanced, good judgement and clear thinking is made possible – when the organ is unbalanced, frustration and clouded judgement will result.

Bladder meridian

The bladder meridian begins at the inside corner of the eye, passes over the forehead and the top of the head, then continues down the back in four lines, two on either side of the spine. The four lines continue over the buttocks and down the legs, where two meet behind each knee. A single line then passes down each leg along the centre line of the calf behind the outer ankle, and ends at the outer tip of the little toe.

Common symptoms of imbalance

Physical

* back problems
* bladder infection
* incontinence
* hip or sacrum problems
* pain on inside corner of eye

* rounded shoulders
* spasm or pain at back of calf
* stiffness in little toe
* aching feet after standing

Emotional

* paranoia
* jealousy
* excessive suspicion

* fear
* chronic anxiety

> ## Key Note
>
> **In Chinese medicine, the bladder is part of the system that includes the kidneys and the reproductive organs. By boosting energy along the bladder meridian, you strengthen not only the bladder itself but every organ in the body.**

Triple warmer meridian

The triple warmer meridian begins on the outside corner of the nail on the fourth finger and runs up the middle of the outside of the arm to the top of the shoulder. It continues over the shoulder to the clavicle, up the back of the neck and circles around the back of the ear, where it continues to the outer corner of the eyebrow.

Common symptoms of imbalance

Physical

* distended abdomen
* colds and fevers
* deafness
* pain behind ear

* elbow problems
* swollen jaw
* slow metabolism, overweight
* fast metabolism, hyperactive

Emotional

* none

Key Note

In Chinese medicine, the triple warmer, also known as the triple heater, does not relate to a specific organ, but is seen as having a function that controls fluids within the body, most specifically water and the endocrine system.

The triple warmer gets its name from the three centres of activity within the body that create heat as they function.

* The upper warmer is associated with the heart and the lungs.
* The middle warmer is associated with the liver, spleen and stomach.
* The lower warmer is associated with the kidneys, bladder, small and large intestines.

Conception vessel meridian

The conception vessel meridian starts in the pelvic cavity, drops down and merges in the perineum just between the anus and the genitals. It then crosses through the genital area to the top of the pubic bone, runs up the midline of the abdomen, chest and neck and ends just below the lower lip.

Common symptoms of imbalance

Physical

* asthma
* coughing
* epilepsy
* eczema
* hay fever
* head and neck pain
* laryngitis

* lung problems
* mouth sores
* pneumonia
* genital disorders
* itching
* painful abdominal skin

Emotional

* none

> **Key Note**
>
> In Chinese medicine, the conception vessel is seen as the regulator of the peripheral nervous system and along with the governing vessel controls the other 12 meridians.
>
> It creates balance by uniting the organ meridians, allowing energy flow to adjust when there is a blockage. In addition to providing energy to all of your peripheral nerves, the conception vessel also governs menstruation and the development of the foetus.

Governing vessel meridian

The governing vessel meridian begins in the pelvic cavity and then drops down and merges below the genital area. It then passes to the tip of the coccyx. From here, it moves upward across the sacrum and along the spine, up over the head towards the upper lip. It then goes under the lip to the upper gum.

Common symptoms of imbalance

Physical

* headaches and pain in the eyes
* stiffness in the spine
* back pain or tension
* dizziness
* eye problems
* cold extremities

* fevers
* haemorrhoids
* insomnia
* neck pain
* spinal problems
* rounded shoulders, heavy head

Emotional

* none

Key Note

In Chinese medicine, the governing vessel is the regulator of the nervous system and, along with the conception vessel, it controls the other 12 meridians.

Like the conception vessel, it allows excess energy to pass through it, which in turn passes that excess on to other meridians that may be deficient of energy.

It is considered as being an extra meridian by the Chinese.

Key Note

When working along a specific meridian, remember that you are also working on a related organ. Meridians are energetic roots or organs. When pressing on a point along a meridian, energy is boosted along the pathway to the corresponding organ.

It is important to realise that emotions can upset the natural balance and flow of electromagnetic energy in the body, by subtly altering the chemical state of the body's tissues and their ionic conductivity.

Yin emotions such as depression, fear, disappointment, grief, withdrawal and shame can cause the body's tissues to be flooded with negative electromagnetic energy. The negative energy that permeates the body's system then causes negative congestion, which deprives the yang circuit and the muscles and tissues supplied by them of positive energy.

Conversely, an excess of yang emotions such as anger, agitation, impatience, frustration, jealousy, hostility, envy and defensiveness can flood the tissues with positive electromagnetic energy, which depletes the yin circuits along with the muscles and tissues supplied by them.

Chakras

Everything that happens to us on an emotional level has an energetic impact on the subtle body, which in turn has an impact on the physical body.

Chakras are non-physical energy centres located about an inch away from the physical body. The energy field of each chakra extends beyond the visible body of matter into the subtle body, or aura.

It is important to remember that chakras do not have a physical form and any illustration of the chakras is merely a visual aid to the imagination and not a literal physical reality.

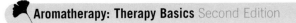

Chakras are a way of describing the flow of subtle energy and are often said to be related to an endocrine gland, which the chakra is thought to influence.

With stress, the chakras can lose their ability to synchronise with each other and become unbalanced.

If negative energy becomes stored in chakras, it can accumulate and the function of the chakra becomes impaired. Ultimately this can lead to energy blocks where the chakra virtually ceases to function and creates an imbalance as other chakras attempt to compensate for the blocked centre, creating additional strain for the energy system.

An accumulation of negative energy in the chakras can manifest itself as an emotional or physical condition. Often we only notice a change in the physical body as we become aware of pain or disease; this may not always be linked to being a symptom of a cause within the subtle body.

Chakras are the focal points for the energies of the subtle bodies and are the key to restoring balancing. By placing hands along the axis of the chakras, energy can be aligned and harmony restored. By working with the subtle energy of the chakras, energy may be strengthened, decreased or balanced as needed by the body at the time of the treatment.

> ## Key Note
>
> **Each essential oil has an affinity with one or more chakras and this information may be used in therapeutic application to strengthen the formulae for helping the client back to balance.**

Base or root chakra

Location: at the base of the spine

Relevance: it is the foundation chakra and is linked with nature and planet Earth. It is concerned with all issues of a physical nature – the body, the senses, sensuality, a person's sex, survival, aggression and self-defence. At a physical level, it is linked to the endocrine system through the adrenal glands. Its energies also affect the lower parts of the pelvis, the hips, legs and feet.

Imbalance: if this chakra is unbalanced it can make a person feel as if they are ungrounded and unfocused. They may feel weak, lack confidence and unable to achieve their goals.

Colour association: red

> ## Key Note
>
> **Examples of essential oils with an affinity for the base chakra include Benzoin, Jasmine and Ylang, Ylang.**

Sacral chakra

Location: at the level of the sacrum between the navel and the base chakra

Relevance: concerned with all issues of creativity and sexuality. At the physical level, it is linked to the testes in the male and the ovaries in the female. Its energies also affect the urino-genital organs, the uterus, the kidneys, the lower digestive organs and the lower back.

Imbalance: a person with an imbalance in this chakra may bury their emotions and be overly sensitive. An imbalance may also lead to sexual difficulties and energy blocks with creativity.

Colour association: orange

Key Note

Examples of essential oils with an affinity for the sacral chakra include Jasmine, Patchouli and Sandalwood.

Solar plexus chakra

Location: at approximately waist level

Relevance: this chakra relates to our emotions, self-esteem and self-worth. Feelings such as fear, anxiety, insecurity, jealousy and anger are generated here. At a physical level, it is linked to the Islets of Langerhans in the pancreas. Its energies also affect the solar and splenic nerve plexuses, the digestive system, the pancreas, liver, gall bladder, diaphragm and middle back.

Imbalance: people who are under a degree of stress will show imbalance in this chakra, as shock and stress impact on this chakra more than others. It is in the solar plexus chakra that negative energies relating to thoughts and feelings are processed. People with an imbalance in this chakra may feel depressed, insecure, lacking in confidence and may worry what others think.

Colour association: yellow

Key Note

Examples of essential oils with an affinity for the solar plexus chakra include Fennel, Grapefruit, Neroli and Petitgrain.

Heart chakra

Location: in the centre of the chest

Relevance: this chakra is concerned with love and the heart. It deals with all issues relating to love and affection. At a physical level it is linked to the thymus gland. Its energies also affect the cardiac and pulmonary nerve plexuses, the heart, lungs, bronchial tubes, chest, upper back and arms.

It is also the point of connection between the upper and lower chakras.

Imbalance: if the energy does not flow freely between the solar plexus and the heart, or between the heart and the throat, it can lead to some form of imbalance due to the energy withdrawal into the body. A person with an imbalance in this chakra may feel sorry for himself or herself, be afraid of letting go, feel unworthy of love or terrified of rejection.

Colour association: green

Key Note

Examples of essential oils with an affinity for the heart chakra include Bergamot, Geranium, Melissa and Rose.

Throat chakra

Location: at the base of the neck

Relevance: this chakra is concerned with communication and expression; it also deals with the issue of truth and true expression of the soul. At a physical level, it is linked to the thyroid and parathyroid glands. Its energies also affect the pharyngeal nerve plexus, the organs of the throat, the neck, nose, mouth, teeth and ears.

Imbalance: if this chakra is out of balance it may result in the inability to express emotions, and as a result of unexpressed feeling bottling up it can lead to frustration and tension. A person with an imbalance in this chakra may feel unable to relax.

Colour association: blue

Key Note

Examples of essential oils with an affinity for the throat chakra include the Chamomiles (Roman and German), Rosemary and Sweet Marjoram.

Brow chakra

Location: in the middle of the forehead over the third eye area

Relevance: commonly known as the 'third eye', the brow chakra is the storehouse of memories and imagination and is associated with intellect, understanding and intuition. At a physical level, it is linked to the hypothalamus and pituitary gland. Its energies also affect the nerves of the head, brain, eyes and face.

Imbalance: if this chakra is not functioning correctly it can lead to headaches and nightmares. A person with an imbalance in this chakra may be oversensitive to others' feelings, afraid of success, non-assertive and undisciplined.

Colour association: indigo

Key Note

Examples of essential oils with an affinity for the brow chakra/third eye include Clove, Rosemary and Teatree.

Crown chakra

Location: on top of the head

Relevance: this chakra is the centre of our spirituality and is concerned with thinking and decision making. At a physical level it is linked to the pineal gland. Its energies also affect the brain and the rest of the body.

Imbalance: an imbalance in this chakra may be reflected in those who are unwilling or afraid to open up to their own spiritual potential. An imbalance may also show as being unable to make decisions.

Colour association: violet

Key Note

Examples of essential oils with an affinity for the crown chakra include Clary Sage, Lavender, Frankincense and Patchouli.

Self-assessment Questions

1. Explain why it is useful for an aromatherapist to have an insight into energy-based concepts in relation to aromatherapy.

----

2. *State the energetic roles of the following:*

   i *Yin and Yang*

----

   ii *Meridians*

----

iii Chakras

----

3. Give an example of how essential oils may be used to help address imbalances in

   i   Yin and Yang

----

   ii Chakras

----

iii Meridians

CHAPTER 10

Aromatherapy Massage and Other Forms of Treatment

Aromatherapy massage represents the earliest form of treatment used in Roman and Egyptian times, and is still the primary form of treatment used in aromatherapy today. It allows the essential oils to be absorbed through the skin to affect the body and treats the body directly by the therapeutic effects of the massage itself.

* A competent aromatherapist needs to be able to prepare for and provide an aromatherapy massage incorporating a range of techniques.

Objectives

By the end of this chapter you will be able to relate the following knowledge to your work as an aromatherapist:

* the benefits of aromatherapy massage
* the range of aromatherapy massage techniques and their effects
* the hygiene and safety involved in preparing for an aromatherapy massage
* relaxation techniques that may be integrated into aromatherapy massage treatments
* types of treatment given and commercial timings
* after-care advice given to a client following aromatherapy massage
* other forms of treatment using essential oils.

An aromatherapy massage has three main benefits:

* It aids absorption of essential oils into the bloodstream.
* There is the psychological benefit of inhaling the vapour itself.
* The massage itself has therapeutic effects and can relax and/or stimulate the client.

Aromatherapy Massage Techniques

Massage is the most important method of application of aromatherapy, as it is the most effective way of introducing essential oils to affect the body systems, and there is the added benefit of therapeutic touch.

Due to the diversity of essential oils and their individual therapeutic properties, the benefits and effects of aromatherapy massage are many:

Psychological benefits

* Enhances a general state of well-being

* Calms and soothes the mind

* Helps reduce nervous tension

* Helps lift the mood and feelings of depression

Physiological benefits

* Enhances lymphatic drainage – helps reduce fluid retention and prevent oedema

* Induces a feeling of deep relaxation in the body

* Helps to restore balance in the body

* Stimulates the body's natural immunity

* Increases the oxygen and nutrient supply to the tissues by increasing the blood circulation

* Can help to increase energy levels as blockages and congestion in the nerves are eased.

There is a wide variety in the massage techniques used by aromatherapists, depending on training and qualifications. However, aromatherapy massage techniques in general comprise the Swedish massage techniques of *effleurage*, *petrissage*, *friction* and *vibrations*, alongside techniques such as *pressure* and *neuromuscular*.

Whatever the method used, the movements used in aromatherapy are generally relaxing movements, omitting the more vigorous techniques such as *tapotement*. The movements are usually performed slowly, in order to induce relaxation and stress relief.

Effleurage
Technique
These are soothing and stroking movements that precede, connect and conclude any massage sequence. They are classified as *superficial* and *deep*.

Effleurage is performed with the palmar surface of the hand and should follow the venous and lymphatic flow. It is usually performed slowly as it is aimed at the slow circulation.

Effects
Effleurage:

* promotes venous flow, thereby increasing and improving general circulation

* increases lymphatic flow; hastens removal and absorption of waste products

* aids desquamation and increases the skin's elasticity

* improves the capillary circulation to the skin and nutrition to the skin's tissues

* provides continuity in the massage by linking other movements

* allows client to become accustomed to the aromatherapist's touch

* has a soothing effect on sensory nerve endings, inducing a state of relaxation
* aids absorption of essential oils into the bloodstream.

Petrissage
Technique
This technique involves lifting the tissues away from the underlying structures and is often generically referred to as *kneading*. Pressure is smoothly and firmly applied and then relaxed. This movement should be performed with supple, relaxed hands that apply intermittent pressure with either one or both hands, or parts of the hands.

Effects
Petrissage:

* increases circulation and hastens elimination of waste from the tissues
* improves the tone and elasticity of muscles due to the increased blood supply
* aids relaxation of tense muscle fibres by carrying away products of fatigue and relieving pain.

Frictions
Technique
These are small movements performed with the pad of the thumb or fingertips. They are small concentrated movements exerting controlled pressure on a small area of the surface tissues, moving them over the underlying structures

Effects
Friction:

* stimulates circulation and metabolism within the tissues
* helps to break down and free skin adhesions
* aids absorption of fluid around joints
* presents the formation of fibrosis in the muscle tissue
* can have an invigorating or relaxing effect.

Vibrations
Technique
These are fine trembling movements performed along a nerve path with one or both hands, using either the palmar surface of the hands or the fingertips.

Effects
Vibrations:

* stimulate and clear nerve pathways
* create a sedative effect, helping to relieve tension and refresh the client.

Neuromuscular
Technique
These are forms of massage techniques that use friction, vibration and pressure movements to help influence nerve pathways and muscles. They can help to release energy blocks by stimulating the nerves.

Effects
Neuromuscular techniques:

* stimulate the nerve supply to the corresponding organ

* stimulate cell renewal

* clear congestion in the nerves

* help to relieve muscular spasms.

Pressures
Technique
These techniques are performed by applying pressures on every inch of the skin with the thumbs or fingers, along the nerve tracts or meridians. These techniques are a form of 'energy' massage.

Effects
Pressures:

* stimulate the nerves and clear energy blocks

* ease congestion in the nervous system by relieving tension from the nerve tracts.

Key Note

The increase in blood flow and warmth created by aromatherapy massage techniques increases the rate of absorption of essential oils into the bloodstream. Massage is therefore a very effective way of enhancing the absorption of oils to affect the systems of the body.

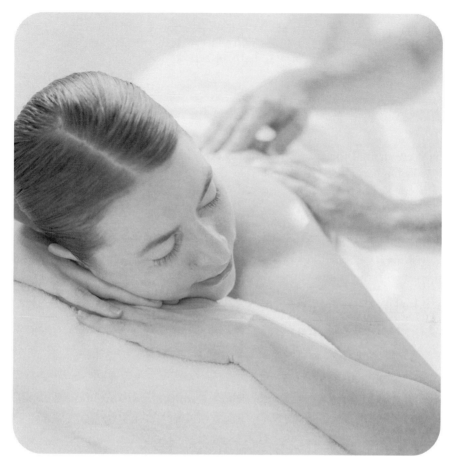

* Photo 38: The psychological and physiological benefits of massage are considerable. *

Preparing for the Aromatherapy Massage

Maintaining employment standards

An aromatherapist should present a smart and hygienic working appearance at all times, in order to project a professional attitude.

As part of maintaining employment standards, aromatherapists should pay particular attention to the following factors:

Clothing

Professional workwear should be worn at all times and should be clean and smart. Remember that the appearance of an aromatherapist can greatly influence a client into using their services on a regular basis.

Footwear

Footwear should be comfortable and clean, and matching the colour of workwear. Shoes should be flat or with a small heel, and enclosed (for hygiene reasons).

Hair

Long hair should be tied back with co-ordinating hair accessories; this is not only hygienic, but practical.

Jewellery

No jewellery should be worn for applying aromatherapy massage other than a wedding band, as jewellery may scratch or irritate a client and has the potential to harbour germs.

Hands

Hands should be kept as soft as possible and protected from harsh chemicals. Nails must be kept short and unvarnished.

Aromatherapists must ensure that they wash their hands very thoroughly before and after each treatment, for hygiene reasons. It is also important to ensure that they do not build up sensitivity to essential oils, resulting in their hands becoming cracked or sore.

Personal hygiene

Due to the close nature of working with aromatherapy, personal hygiene is of paramount importance. It is also important to avoid wearing strong smelling aftershaves and perfumes, as this may not only be offensive to the client but could interact with the aroma of the essential oils.

Preparation of the treatment area for aromatherapy

The treatment area should always look hygienically clean and tidy, but also comfortable and not too clinical. This can be achieved by giving thought to the following factors:

Lighting

This should be soft and discreet; try to avoid overhead lights, which are glaring and not conducive to relaxation.

Ventilation

Ensure that the treatment area is well ventilated and draught free. It is advisable to air the room regularly between clients, by opening windows, to ensure the atmosphere remains fresh and that the build of aromas in the room is not too overpowering – this could make you or your client feel nauseous.

Temperature

This should be comfortably warm (approximately 70–75 degrees).

Decor and colours

Colouring should be chosen carefully as some colours are warm, whilst others will feel too cold and clinical. Towels should preferably match the decor and add to the warmth of the room.

Privacy

A treatment area should always be private to ensure client relaxation.

Atmosphere and noise level

Creating a relaxing atmosphere is a very important requirement of the aromatherapy massage, which can be aided by using a relaxation tape. Always ensure before you commence the aromatherapy massage, that you will not be disturbed by anyone entering the treatment room or a ringing phone.

Health, Safety and Hygiene

As aromatherapy massage is a personalised treatment and there is close contact between the client and aromatherapist, there is a specific need to avoid cross-infection. In order to ensure health and safety, consideration should be given to:

* the treatment area and equipment used

* the client

* the aromatherapist

The treatment area

In order to adhere to all health, safety and hygiene requirements, attention must be paid to the following:

* Keep the treatment area hygienically clean at all times.

* Keep the area free from obstructions.

* Ensure that all equipment is regularly disinfected.

* Ensure all floor coverings are slip-proof.

* Install hand-washing facilities in the vicinity of the treatment area.

* Dispose of all rubbish in a lined and covered bin; empty at regular intervals.

* Ensure all equipment is stable and fit for use by checking all hinges and locks.

* Maintain all electrical equipment regularly by having it checked by a qualified engineer once a year.

* Be familiar with the location and the correct usage of fire extinguishers.

* Clearly indicate all fire exits and fire evacuation procedures.

* Keep a well-maintained first-aid kit in the treatment area.

* Store all product equipment correctly and safely.

* Ensure the correct maintenance of heating and ventilation systems.

The client

* Check client for contra-indications to ensure they are suitable for treatment.

* Use clean towels and disposable tissue covering, for each client.

* Wash hands before and after each client to avoid cross-infection.

* Check the client for any contagious or infectious disorders.

* Ensure client has removed all jewellery.

* Avoid open wounds and sores and ensure they are covered with a waterproof plaster.

* Do not give an aromatherapy massage if you are ill or contagious.

* Check client's skin type before treatment; if necessary, do a skin test to avoid skin irritation and sensitisation resulting from the incorrect use of essential oils.

* Help clients on and off the massage couch.

* Ensure client is hygienically prepared for treatment by showering to remove all perfumes and cosmetics, wearing a suitable head covering if hair is long and that they retain their pants.

The aromatherapist

∗ Present a smart and hygienic appearance at all times.

∗ Always wear professional workwear.

∗ Cover all cuts or abrasions with a waterproof plaster.

∗ Avoid cross-infection by using disposable spatulas to remove any products; keep lids tightly on bottles.

∗ Use correct lifting techniques when moving equipment.

∗ Use correct posture and stance when carrying out aromatherapy massage.

∗ Use equipment and products in accordance with manufacturers' instructions.

∗ Wash hands thoroughly before and after each client.

∗ Maintain first-aid skills.

∗ Know the location of the first-aid kit and fire evacuation procedures.

∗ Be familiar with the fire-fighting equipment.

∗ Be familiar with contra-indications so as to know when a client may be treated and when they should be referred to a medical practitioner.

Relaxation Techniques

There are several relaxation techniques that may be used to assist a client to relax before, during and after their aromatherapy massage:

Meditation

This is a very effective method of relaxation, as the idea is to focus thoughts on relaxing for a period of time, leaving the mind and body to recover from the problems and worries that have caused the stress.

Meditation can help to reduce stress by slowing down breathing, helping muscular relaxation, reducing blood pressure, and helping to clear thinking by focusing and concentrating the mind.

The key to meditation is to quieten the mind and focus completely on one thing. It is important for the body to be relaxed and in a comfortable position.

Meditation is a very personal experience and can involve a person sitting or lying quietly and focusing the mind, or can be taught in a class situation. Therapists may also facilitate meditation by using positive mental imagery and visualisation in order to help clients focus their mind on their imagery and lift themselves into a state of passive awareness in order to relax.

Breathing

Deep breathing is a very effective method of relaxation and works well combined with other relaxation techniques such as relaxation imagery, meditation and progressive muscular relaxation.

Breathing is affected when people experience physical or emotional stress. During times of stress, breathing becomes shallow and irregular, resulting in the brain being deprived of sufficient oxygen, leading to feelings of dizziness, inability to concentrate and agitation.

Deep breathing fills the body with positive energy and clears the mind and can therefore prevent people from getting stressed or can help them gain control more quickly when they feel stressed.

Breathing exercise 1

1 Sit or lie in a comfortable position and loosen tight clothing.

2 Place one hand on the chest and the other across the stomach.

3 Inhale deeply through the nose to fill the upper chest cavity and down to the lower part of the lungs, as if breathing into the stomach, for a count of 6.

4 Exhale slowly to a count of 12, allowing the air to escape from the top of your lungs first before the lower part deflates.

5 Repeat this exercise 6–8 times.

Breathing exercise 2

1 Apply the first two fingers of the right hand to the side of the right nostril and press gently to close it. Breathe in slowly through the left nostril and hold for a count of 3.

2 Transfer the first two fingers to the left nostril to close it.

3 Breathe out slowly through the right nostril on a count of 3. Breathe in through the right nostril and hold for a count of 3 and whilst holding transfer the fingers to the right nostril and breathe out through the left nostril.

4 Repeat the exercise 6 times.

Correct breathing is something that really needs to be practised often until it feels natural and it may then be utilised as a counterbalance to stress. Breathing properly enables the body to relax and regain its natural balance, whilst calming the mind.

If a client has difficulty breathing correctly, it may be advisable for them to attend classes that involve structured breathing, such as yoga.

Progressive muscular relaxation (PMR)

This is a physical technique, designed to relax the body when it is tense. It may be applied to any group of muscles in the body, depending on whether one area or the whole body is tense.

PMR is achieved by tensing a group of muscles so that they are as tightly contracted as possible. The muscles are then held in a state of tension for a few seconds and relaxed. This should result in a feeling of deep relaxation in the muscles.

For maximum effect, this exercise should be combined with breathing exercises and imagery, such as the image of stress leaving the body.

Relaxation exercise

1 Find a place where you can feel comfortable.

2 Close your eyes and pull your feet towards you as far as you can and then hold them for a count of 5 and then let them relax. Let them drop as if you are a puppet on a string and the string has broken.

3 Curl your toes as if you were holding a pencil and hold them for a count of 5 and then relax.

4 Tighten and tense the calf muscles, count to 5 and then relax.

5 Tighten and tense the thighs, press them tightly together, count to 5 and then relax, allowing them to fall apart.

6 Tighten the abdominal muscles, pulling in the muscles, count to 5 and then relax.

7 Tighten the muscles in the hips and the buttocks, count to 5 and then relax.

8 Arch the back and tense the back muscles, count to 5 and then relax.

9 Tense the shoulders by raising them to the ears, count to 5 and then drop them.

10 Lift your arms up with the hands outstretched as if you were reaching for something. Hold for a slow count of 5 and then let the arms drop down.

11 Tense the muscles in the forehead, count to 5 and then relax.

12 Tense the muscles around the eyes tightly, count to 5 and then relax.

13 Tense the muscles in the jaw and cheeks (as if gritting your teeth), hold to a count of 5 and then relax.

14 By now you should feel relaxed and heavy, as if you are sinking into the floor or chair. Check that all body parts are free from tension and, if there are any areas left with tension, hold that part tense again before relaxing.

15 When you're ready, get up gradually, taking your time.

Note: This exercise will be easier to do if the instructions are on tape, preferably spoken by a person with a slow, calm and relaxing voice.

Imagery and visualisation

Imagery techniques can be useful to recreate a retreat from stress and pressure, by remembering a place or event that was happy and restful and calling upon it to help manage a stressful period.

Imagery and visualisation is often more effective and real if it is combined with sounds, smell, taste and warmth, for instance, imagining being on a beach, with the warmth of the sun, the water lapping on the shore.

Imagery and visualisation can often be enhanced by a relaxation tape; there are several on the market that are designed specifically for aromatherapy massage.

Aromatherapy Massage Procedure

There are three main forms of treatment offered in aromatherapy massage. The choice will depend on the client's needs and preference, and most probably the cost.

* Full aromatherapy massage usually takes between 1 hour, and 1 hour and 15 minutes.

* Full aromatherapy massage including the face and scalp usually takes 1 and a half hours.

* Part body aromatherapy massage applied locally to body parts usually takes between 30 and 45 minutes, depending on which areas are treated.

> ## Key Note
>
> Whatever method of treatment is given, it is essential that it is adapted to suit the individual needs of the client. A client's needs will vary from treatment to treatment, and there may be a need to change the previous treatment plan due to a change in the client's condition or circumstances.
>
> It is also important to ensure that the treatment given is cost-effective in terms of time.

Before the massage

Follow these guidelines to ensure a safe and effective aromatherapy massage:

* Carry out a consultation to identify whether the client is unsuitable for treatment, and check for contra-indications.
* Complete records; check that the client agrees with the information and signs the declaration.
* Assess client needs to establish the objectives of the treatment.
* Formulate a treatment plan with the client: the treatment objectives, the treatment method and the time it will take.
* Select and blend oils ready for use, and ask client to approve the selection.
* Check that all necessary working materials are to hand and the treatment area and couch have been correctly prepared with clean towels and tissues.
* Advise the client to empty their bladder and disrobe ready for treatment.
* Ensure client is warm, comfortable and relaxed before treatment commences.

> ## Key Note
>
> If the face and scalp are to be included in the treatment, you will need to ensure that the client's face has been cleansed and is free from cosmetics and make-up before treatment.

After-care advice

The following advice should be given to a client following aromatherapy massage:

* **Avoid skin washing and bathing** for approximately eight hours after treatment as this will enable the essential oils to fully penetrate the skin and have their effects on the body through the bloodstream. Most

essential oils can take up to 60 minutes to be absorbed through the skin and can carry out their therapeutic work for up to eight hours afterwards.

* **Avoid direct exposure to strong sunlight** following the use of any phototoxic oils.

* **Avoid alcohol and smoking:** it is important for a client not to smoke or drink for at least 24 hours after treatment as aromatherapy massage is a detoxifying treatment.

* **Drink plenty of fresh water and herbal infusions:** as aromatherapy is essentially a cleansing treatment, drinking plenty of water and herbal teas can assist in the elimination of toxins from the body and help the healing process.

* **Eat a light diet:** it is important to eat a light and natural diet as the body needs to concentrate its effort on detoxification and natural healing. Fresh and natural foods are advisable, because over-refined and processed food adds to the toxicity of the body.

* **Enjoy rest and relaxation:** in order to assist the healing process, the client should be advised to rest as much as possible following treatment. Clients will invariably feel tired after treatment and they will benefit from a good rest. The feeling of tiredness will often be replaced by a feeling of vitality.

Post-aromatherapy massage procedure

* Allow the client to rest while you wash your hands thoroughly to remove all residue of oils.

* Offer client a glass of water.

* Allow client to change and help them off the couch.

* Offer client after-care advice.

* Evaluate the effectiveness of the treatment by gaining feedback from the client. Ask how they are feeling and whether treatment has been successful in meeting the overall treatment objectives.

* Review the treatment plan with the client.

* Make recommendations for a future treatment and book the client's next appointment.

* Complete treatment records ensuring that you have kept an accurate record of essential oils used, dates and results.

Key Note

In order to enhance the effects of the massage, aromatherapists may wish to make up individual bath oils for clients to use at home. Remember that all blends given to clients must be clearly labelled, with their contents, amounts used and the date blended. It is also advisable to include an expiry date.

Task

In order to gain as much experience in aromatherapy as possible, carry out several case studies that involve many clients having aromatherapy massage treatments over a period of time.

Try to select as wide a range of clients as possible both in terms of age and condition. After undertaking a full consultation with them:

* formulate and agree a treatment plan
* perform aromatherapy massage techniques over a period of time, using a range of aromatherapy massage movements
* evaluate the effectiveness of the treatments
* advise the client on after-care and home-care procedures.

Other Forms of Treatment

Although massage should always be the primary form of treatment, there are instances when it may be inappropriate or when other forms of treatment may be used to enhance the effectiveness of treatment.

Aromatic baths

This method is effective for clients' self-use and may be used between treatments to reinforce the treatment given by the aromatherapist.

Method

Essential oils may be added directly to the bath water or blended in carrier oil first. If adding the essential oils directly to the water, take care to disperse in the water as the oils will not dilute in the water, but will float on the top.

A safe amount of essential oil to add to the bath is up to **six** drops of most oils. *Note:* Oils such as *Lemon* and *Peppermint* need to be restricted to **two** or **three** drops only, as they could cause adverse skin reactions if used to excess. Certain essential oils such as *Clove* and *Cinnamon* are unsuitable for use in the bath as they are skin irritants.

Key Note

Never use undiluted oils in the bath for babies, young children and those with sensitive skin: always dilute them in a carrier oil first.

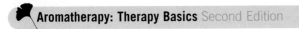

If making up an aromatic bath oil for a client, the same dilution rate of 2 per cent essential oil to carrier oil applies. Always ensure you have labelled the blend and that you have instructed the client on self-use. Usually one or two capfuls will be sufficient for a bath with the recommended treatment time of 15–20 minutes.

Hand and foot baths

These can be useful to treat areas that cannot be massaged, for example an arthritic or otherwise injured limb.

Method

The amount of essential oils would be restricted to two–four drops for a hand bath and two–six drops for a foot bath, depending on the choice of oils.

The hands and feet are highly penetrative areas and, if someone cannot be obviously treated with massage, then it is a useful way of absorbing the oils into the bloodstream for therapeutic benefit.

Steam inhalation

This method is especially suited to sinus, throat and chest infections.

Method

A single drop may be enough, and four drops is the maximum. Try one drop only the first time: **do not inhale for longer than about 60 seconds at a time if you have a history of asthma or allergies**.

Provided this is well tolerated, you can then increase the amount of oil used and lengthen the treatment time to five minutes or more.

Compresses

This is a very effective way of using essential oils to relieve pain and reduce inflammation.

Method

A *hot compress* may be made by filling a bowl with very hot water and then adding four or five drops of essential oil (depending on the oil). Dip a piece of absorbent material such as cotton wool or a flannel or lint into the water, squeeze out the excess and then place over the affected area until it has cooled, then repeat. Hot compresses are particularly useful for backache, rheumatism, arthritis, abscesses, earache and toothache.

Cold compresses are made in a similar way, using ice-cold rather than hot water and these are useful for headaches, sprains, strains and hot, swollen conditions.

Burners and vaporisers

This method is used for vaporising essential oils in a room. The simplest form of *burner* involves a night light and a section that is filled with water.

Method

Up to 12 drops of essential oil may be added to the water section of the burner. The heat of the night light evaporates the water and the essential oil, vaporising the odour into the atmosphere.

Another way of diffusing essential oils into the atmosphere involves a small heating element and a small pad onto which the drops of essential oil are placed – this is more commonly known as a *vaporiser*.

Blending with creams

Essential oils may be blended into base creams for client self-application, as the client may find it easier and more convenient to apply a cream or lotion as part of their home-care treatment.

Method

* Take an unperfumed cream or lotion.
* Add any special carriers to the cream/lotion first, a little at a time, and mix well.
* Fill the pot or jar with three-quarters of the required cream/lotion and then add the essential oils and shake well.
* Add the rest of the cream/lotion and leave a 10 per cent air gap to ensure an even blend of oils.
* Label and ensure you have given the client clear instructions for self-application.

Base creams or lotions may be bought from good essential oil suppliers. They should be unperfumed and made from pure and natural plant substances.

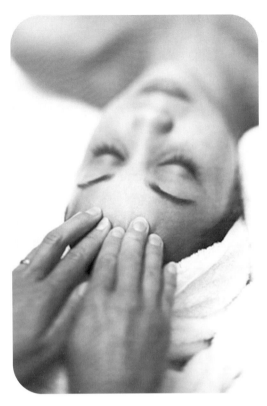

✳ Photo 39: Massage to the head ✳

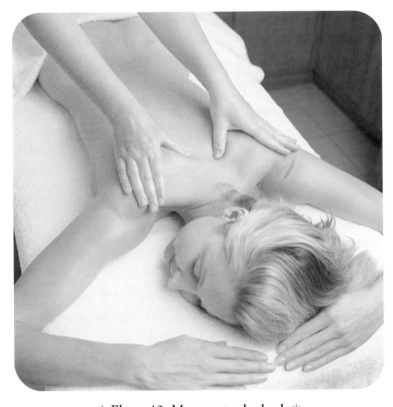

✳ Photo 40: Massage to the back ✳

Self-assessment Questions

1. Why is massage one of the most effective ways of absorbing essential oils into the bloodstream for therapeutic effect?

----

2. Describe the effects of the following movements used in aromatherapy massage:

   i   effleurage

----

   ii   neuromuscular

----

iii pressures

----

3. State five important health and safety factors when preparing the treatment area for aromatherapy massage.

----

4 State five important health and safety factors when preparing the client for aromatherapy massage.

----

5. What general after-care advice should be offered to a client following an aromatherapy massage and why?

CHAPTER 11
Basic Business Skills for the Aromatherapist

As complementary therapies continue to grow in popularity, more and more business opportunities are developing that will enable therapists to practise aromatherapy professionally.

Whether self-employed, managing a business, or working as an employee, it is very important to be able to understand and implement good business practice.

* A competent aromatherapist needs to be able to understand the principles of business management in order to be successful and ensure the smooth running of a business.

Objectives

By the end of this chapter you will be able to relate the following to your work as an aromatherapist:

* maintaining employment standards for commercial practice

* the requirements for setting up an aromatherapy practice

* marketing and advertising

* professional ethics

* professional associations.

In order to run a successful aromatherapy practice, it is important not only to be good at the skill you practise but also to develop good business skills that will help you to maintain *and* develop your business.

Being a good aromatherapist is not enough to ensure a successful business. One of the main reasons that small businesses fail at an early stage is due to poor management.

A successful business depends on

* a good image

* a good reputation

* a high degree of professionalism

* sufficient resources to deliver a quality service

* effective record keeping.

Maintaining Employment Standards

There are several important factors to take into account when working as an aromatherapist in order to maintain and monitor the standard of service you offer to clients.

It is important not only to perform a skill competently but to be able to apply it in a commercially acceptable way.

Aromatherapists must bear in mind at all times that they are part of the service industry, and the following factors could affect the day-to-day running and the overall efficiency of the business:

* communication skills
* management and staff responsibilities
* working conditions
* establishment rules and quality assurance
* record keeping
* resources – planning and monitoring.

Communication skills

Whether a sole trader or a large business, a successful business relies on good communication. Communication skills are extremely important when there are several colleagues working together in the same clinic, and information needs to be conveyed and received.

If communications skills are broken down for as little as half an hour in a busy clinic, it can have a very dramatic effect on the service given and the overall efficiency and image of the clinic. Good communication means being able to liaise well with clients, colleagues and other visitors who may enter or telephone the clinic, such as a supplier or another fellow professional.

Communication skills may be used to:

* identify clients' needs
* inform clients about a service
* inform clients and colleagues of changes in procedures
* maintain workplace records

Communication may involve:

* talking
* listening
* writing
* eye contact
* body language.

When communicating with clients or colleagues over the telephone or in person, it is very important to have good *listening* skills, to ensure that you have received the information they are trying to convey to you correctly.

It is very important to *clarify* what a client has said before acting on it, to ensure that you have received the right information. It is equally important that, when you are speaking to a client or a colleague, you *speak clearly* and accurately to ensure that everything has been understood.

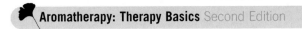

It is most important that *non-verbal* signs that you send out reflect what you are saying. Non-verbal signs are usually picked up from posture, facial expressions and gestures. Try to use effective *body language*, so that you appear friendly and approachable, even when you are not speaking.

Eye contact is very important when talking and listening. Remember that your personal presentation will make a lasting impression, so you should project a professional image from the start.

Written communication

An efficient working environment providing services such as aromatherapy to clients relies on accurate, legible record keeping, which is kept up to date. Records may either be computer based or hand written.

Written communication may involve the recording of messages to colleagues to ensure continuity of service, or the completion of client records in the workplace to ensure therapeutic continuity.

In the workplace, it is very important that all messages are recorded accurately to ensure continuity of operation and services.

Written communication should be clear, dated and timed, along with the action required. It should also be positioned where the person it is intended for will notice it.

Client records should be completed fully, accurately and legibly at the time of the treatment.

Responding to clients' requests

As clients are at the centre of every business it is essential for therapists to respond to their requests promptly, accurately and enthusiastically. Requests for information may come from a telephone enquiry, a personal caller to the workplace or may be in the form of a written request.

It is important to assume a friendly and approachable manner when dealing with clients' requests and use phrases such as 'How may I help you?' It is also important to provide accurate information on treatments such as

* the benefits of the services
* the cost (of individual and courses of treatment)
* the treatment duration
* any pre-treatment advice (such as not wearing body lotions and perfumes before an aromatherapy massage)
* how often the client should attend for maximum benefit.

Maintaining effective relationships with colleagues

A successful business depends on a good image and reputation, but also on the way in which staff work together as a team to maintain the image and professionalism of the establishment. Working with colleagues as a team helps enhance smooth operations and promotes a pleasant working environment and a friendly atmosphere.

Working as a team involves:

* building a good rapport with each other
* understanding each other's responsibilities
* working efficiently within your own job responsibilities
* responding to each other's requests politely and co-operatively

* providing support and assistance, when required
* working together for the needs of the business.

Communication is essential when working with others in a team, and regular meetings can help to maintain effective working relationships.

Meetings provide an opportunity to:

* identify and resolve problems in the workplace
* avoid breakdown in communication and misunderstandings
* contribute and exchange ideas on how workplace practices may be enhanced
* identify training needs
* maintain good working relationships

Establishment rules

An aromatherapist should understand that their work activities and responsibilities must comply with the rules of the establishment in which they are working. Establishment rules lay down a benchmark of standards required by the workplace and are set according to the requirements of the individual business.

In the workplace, aromatherapists have a responsibility to their manager or supervisor, to their clients and to their colleagues.

The responsibilities of an aromatherapist to a supervisor are to ensure that they:

* adhere to the establishment's rules
* understand and adhere to legislation in relation to the provision of services
* report any hazard or potential danger observed in the workplace
* have a sincere commitment to provide a high standard of work to enhance the reputation and image of the establishment
* carry out work practices with honesty and integrity
* complete records fully and accurately
* work within their own initiative to make best use of time at work
* provide a high standard of work to ensure client satisfaction and repeat business
* create a good working relationship with other colleagues to enhance a good working environment
* avoid wastage of resources
* make recommendations for improvement in workplace practices, where appropriate
* understand how their job role contributes to the success of the business.

The responsibilities of an aromatherapist to a client are to:

* treat clients with dignity and respect
* respond to clients' requests politely and efficiently
* accurately inform clients of the services provided by the establishment
* provide treatment only when there is a reasonable expectation that it will be advantageous to the client

* take appropriate measures to protect the client's right to privacy and confidentiality

* provide a high standard of service to ensure client satisfaction and the fostering of repeat business

* make recommendations for future treatments that would benefit the client

* make recommendations for home care products that may help their condition.

The responsibilities of an aromatherapist to their colleagues are to:

* create a good working environment by being friendly, helpful and approachable

* share responsibilities fairly to enhance a good team spirit

* ensure good communication channels by passing on messages promptly and recording messages accurately

* inform others of any changes in establishment procedure.

Work conditions

Work conditions should ensure maximum satisfaction to both clients and staff, and are dependent on the following factors:

* the working environment (heating, lighting, ventilation)

* equipment and materials (sufficient in quality and quantity to carry out work to a client's satisfaction and in a commercially acceptable time)

* procedures – these are set by the management; all staff should be aware of the necessary work procedures to enhance smooth running of the clinic.

Draw up a list of a salon clinic manager's duties.

Task

Quality assurance

Every business, however small, should have a quality assurance policy in order to ensure their services and operation are conducted in a systematic way. Quality assurance policies help to monitor the quality and standard of the service provided and are useful in analysing whether the client's needs are met efficiently, effectively and consistently.

Effective ways of monitoring quality assurance include:

* examining workplace practices and how they relate to client needs and the needs of the business

* avoiding complacency, and continuing professional development

* distributing client satisfaction questionnaires

* introducing a client suggestions box

* implementing changes based on recommendations from clients and staff.

Encouraging communication with clients on a regular basis can help to monitor the quality assurance policy of the establishment.

Efficient work practices – cost-effectiveness

Efficient work practice requires an aromatherapist to perform a skill to the required standard of the establishment and the industry, and in a time that is considered to be commercially acceptable.

Cost-effectiveness in terms of the workplace means maintaining treatment times and minimising waste in order to avoid loss of revenue for the establishment. Aromatherapists need to be aware that by adhering to their appointment times and avoiding wastage they are helping to preserve the business's precious resources and thereby helping to maintain their security of employment.

Record keeping

Maintaining accurate and legible client records is both a legal and professional requirement. It helps the aromatherapist to:

* establish an appropriate treatment plan for the client
* identify special cautions and contra-indications associated with the client's condition
* monitor the client's progress
* protect against a legal claim.

Key Note

It is essential for aromatherapists to take care in what they record in their clients' notes/records. Under the Access to Health Records Act 1990, clients have a right of access to any manually stored health records made since November 1991.

It is therefore important to avoid subjective, judgemental or stereotypical phrases and to avoid making references to medical conditions.

An efficient clinic relies on accurate, legible record keeping, which is kept up to date and may be either hand-written or computer-based. Record keeping includes keeping accurate client records, stock records and any other records of importance, such as an accident book. If clients' records are held on a computer it is a legal requirement to register with the Data Protection Agency.

An important factor to remember with client records is to maintain client confidentiality. All records should be kept in a secure environment, and a client's personal details should never be left lying around for anyone to read.

Stock records and simple accounts records are an essential part of the day-to-day running of the business. They should be done regularly so that you may keep a control on the financial resources of the business.

Resources

Resources are the means by which you conduct your business. Resources must be **planned**, **monitored** and **controlled** to ensure that you stay in business. The planning, monitoring and controlling of resources involves a combination of the following:

Staff

Adequate staff resources are essential to a successful business. The optimum situation is to have the maximum staff available at the busy times and the minimum in the quiet times. Staff cost money and their time must be used efficiently. If they are not earning money for the business, consideration must be given to what they can do in the quiet times to promote business.

Information

Planning and monitoring resources involves good communication between clients and colleagues. It is essential that staff are aware of resources, and how they can be controlled by minimising waste and being cost-effective. Staff may also contribute to the planning by indicating to the manager that stock is low and needs to be reordered, or even suggesting a new supplier who is more efficient and economical.

Staff must also be well informed about treatments available in the clinic, so that they can provide information to prospective clients and sell the service effectively.

Materials

This involves all items of stock and consumables used in the clinic. An accurate record should be kept of all stock in the clinic, in a stock control book. Stock records are essential, to ensure that there is adequate stock at all times and to avoid being faced with a disappointed client if you find that you do not have the materials to do the job.

It is equally important not to be over-stocked, as you will be tying up any available capital and stock will deteriorate with age, particularly essential oils and carrier oils, which are subject to degradation.

Stock checks are ideally carried out in accordance with the level of business conducted; weekly or fortnightly if a large volume of stock is being used, or otherwise monthly stocks checks may be sufficient.

Equipment

These are the tools required to perform the treatments you offer. Equipment should be regularly checked and serviced and a record should be kept of this.

Treatments must be planned to ensure cost-effectiveness, taking account of *money, time* and *services*.

Finance

Controlling finance is essential to an efficient business. A daily cash book is important, as this keeps a daily record of all financial transactions.

It is vital to keep a close eye on your accounts and your profit margin, and to look at ways in which you can save money, without cutting down on quality.

You will need to have a short-term and/or long-term financial plan. Short-term planning may involve an overdraft to get you out of a difficult patch, and for the long term you may require a loan to accommodate future plans.

Time

Timing is an essential factor to consider, so that you:

* avoid keeping other clients waiting

* minimise potential inconvenience to a client

* ensure a cost-effective treatment.

Services

These are the services or treatments you offer to a client in the clinic, which must be accurate in terms of information provided, and take account of consumer legislation, as well as customer requirements.

Business Planning

Running a successful business involves an incredible amount of planning. In the long term, the time spent planning will help to create more business and save you from wasting valuable money, time and resources.

No matter how efficient or successful a business, every service can be improved, even if only in a small way; every business should involve short-term and long-term planning.

> **Task**
>
> **Prepare an outline of a Research and Operational Business Plan for starting a new business in aromatherapy, or for improving an existing business by adding aromatherapy.**
>
> **Take account of the factors detailed below, which will form a basis for the points to consider.**

Research plan

Formulating a research plan is essential when considering starting your own business as it enables you to assess the *potential* of the project, along with its costs and estimated income. There are certain costs associated with a new business, which may include the following:

* rent or lease
* utilities (electricity, lighting)
* equipment and supplies
* furniture
* decorating
* stationery and printing
* advertising
* insurance
* legal and professional fees.

There are many factors to consider when formulating a research plan:

Client requirements

* Decide what client market you are aiming at and the individual needs of those clients.
* Ask yourself whether their needs will be met by your service and available resources.
* Carry out some market research by formulating surveys and questionnaires, to assess the need for your service in your area.

Premises

An important consideration for an aromatherapist is where to offer their services; the various options need to be considered with potential clients in mind as well as their own needs.

For each work setting there are advantages and disadvantages and these should be considered carefully. Due to the diversity of aromatherapy practices it is possible to combine renting space in a clinic with home visiting or working from home.

It is important to seek expert legal and professional advice before entering into an agreement, and especially when leasing or buying premises. As these involve considerable expense, it is wise to build an established clientele before considering such a commitment.

Advantages of working from home

* Overheads are low
* No travelling expenses
* Flexible working hours
* Can make good use of time in between clients

Disadvantages of working from home

* Difficulty in separating work from home life due to the environment
* Possible safety risk with strangers
* Requires a high level of commitment and self-discipline

Advantages of home visiting

* Reduces overheads
* Provides the aromatherapist with a flexible working approach
* Can reach clients who would otherwise be unable to use the service

Disadvantages of home visiting

* More time-consuming due to the travelling time/setting up
* Need to be highly organised to ensure cost-effectiveness

Advantages of renting space in a salon/clinic

* Opportunity to work with and network with other professionals
* The salon/clinic will already have an established clientele (a captive audience)
* Costs and resources may be shared (e.g. reception, advertising, rent, etc.)

Disadvantages of renting space in a salon/clinic

* Rent is beyond individual therapist's control and is subject to increases
* Resources and furnishings may not be to liking
* Appointments and enquiries may be dealt with by others

* Overheads may be high
* May not be room for expansion

Advantages of leasing/buying premises

* Complete control over where to practise
* Freedom to develop business as you want
* Room for expansion
* Can let space to other practitioners to share costs

Disadvantages of leasing/buying premises

* More risks involved – high capital investment required
* A considerable amount of time needs to be allocated to managing the finances, and controlling resources and generating income as well as practising
* A high level of commitment and motivation is required

Catchment area

Look into the catchment area and decide who your potential customers are. You may also wish to consider the competition in your catchment area, and how your service will differ from theirs.

Specialist advice

Consider what professional help you will need in setting up your business, and perhaps enlist the help of a business advisor, accountant or solicitor.

Banks and Local Enterprise Agencies, as well as Business Link services (a government incentive run locally) are all a useful source of reference where a considerable amount of support is available to help small businesses.

Legal requirements

Consider what legal requirements you will need to take account of to ensure good commercial practice, and what legislation (local and national) is relevant to your business.

Finance

What finance do you have available, to inject into the business? Will it be self-financed or externally financed? Look at the advantages and disadvantages of short-term (overdrafts) and long-term finance (loans).

Equipment

What equipment and materials will you need to carry out the plan, and how much will it all cost? What stock will you need and in what quantity? Make a list of all expenditure, so that you may assess the starting-up costs.

Operational plan

An operational plan is the next stage from the research plan, as it sets out the actual *running* of the business.

You will need to take account of the following:

* **What services do you intend to offer?** Draw up a price list that includes a detailed description of the treatments on offer, the price and the time allocated to each treatment.

✳ **Which hours of business do you intend to operate?** Consider what times clients will be available to use your services, in order to maximise your business opportunity.

✳ **What price do you intend to charge for the services?** The prices you charge will be dependent on the market, competition, catchment area and your individual overheads. Remember that the service you offer is unique to you and therefore you must value it first in order to put a price on your service. Consider how much you intend to earn and what the potential income of the business is, by considering the income against the expenditure.

✳ **What staff will you need and at what times?** If you are a sole trader, you may just require an answer-phone to take your messages when you are busy with clients, or you may wish to employ a receptionist to book your appointments.

✳ **How do you intend to advertise your services?** Consider the different ways in which you can inform clients of your services.

✳ **What can you do to ensure good public relations and a good professional image?** Consider the ways in which you can project a good public image through your business.

✳ **How will you ensure quality assurance?** Consider how you can improve on customer service and enhance client satisfaction.

✳ **What will you need to protect your business interests?** Consider the types of insurance required for your business in the event of any loss. Comply with any legal or professional association requirements.

There are many different aspects to marketing, but the aim is always the same: to attract clients who will want to buy what you have to offer.

As aromatherapy is a very personal service, it is important to work on the direct approach to marketing and promotion as this is relatively free and often the most effective!

The direct approach to marketing and promotion of aromatherapy
Personal recommendation/word of mouth
This is the most valuable form of advertising for personal treatments like aromatherapy. Once an aromatherapist has established a reputation for excellent customer service and quality skills, a satisfied client will automatically recommend the service to another potential client.

It is important for aromatherapists to be positive about what they do as self-confidence is one of the best marketing tools. Positive enthusiasm is infectious and even if the person you are speaking to does not need the information they may pass it on to someone who does.

The power of the spoken word is very effective in the marketing of services.

Talks and demonstrations
Talks and demonstrations are an effective way of stimulating interest and generating potential clients and targeted groups and they usually work best when presented together.

Talks should be informative and educational in nature (they should tell potential clients how aromatherapy will benefit them). There is a wide range of client groups aromatherapy can help and a demonstration will help to introduce the target audience to the benefits and effects, and will also help to break down barriers or pre-conceptions they may hold about the therapy.

It is useful to identify the needs of the target audience prior to the presentation, as it gives the aromatherapist the advantage of being able to personalise the session. Talks and demonstrations are better when limited to a maximum of 30–40 minutes, with time left to answer questions and to distribute business cards and literature.

The focus of the talk should be about identifying and providing solutions to the clients' needs.

A useful checklist when preparing for talks is to:

* find out as much as possible about the target group before the talk
* confirm the number of people that will be attending
* check out the venue and its suitability
* plan out the talk with a basic outline format
* have a plentiful supply of literature to hand out
* prepare a list of possible questions you may be asked, and specimen answers
* take some relaxation music to help create a relaxing ambience
* aim to involve the audience in the session (encourage questions or use of them to demonstrate on)
* arrive early to plan the room layout and set up
* take your appointment book with you!

Tips when giving talks to the public include:

* rehearsing the material to be used beforehand (know your subject)
* use appropriate language (avoid jargon or words that are too technical)
* speak clearly and confidently (smile)
* make eye contact with the audience
* plan your talk carefully so there is a clear start, middle and end
* summarise and repeat the key points of the talk
* allow sufficient time for questions
* use visual aids to stimulate interest.

Local exhibitions

Exhibitions are an effective way to communicate with lots of potential clients in one place. It is a useful way of distributing brochures and leaflets and of persuading new clients to watch a demonstration of a new service and sample it. When exhibiting it is important to ensure that it is the right type of show for the image of the business or therapist, and to speak to people who have attended the exhibition previously in order to gain feedback from them.

In order to project the right image at an exhibition it is important to ensure that:

* the stand is accessible and situated to your best advantage
* staff on the stand look warm and welcoming, and are approachable to talk to
* the stand looks attractive, neat and tidy
* there is space for people to browse without feeling intimidated, and space to demonstrate the skills you are promoting.

It is also important, if possible, to take the names and contact numbers of those who visited the stand in order that you may contact them after the exhibition.

Building a referral network

This is one of the most successful and inexpensive ways of creating new business.

Current satisfied clients are one of the most effective means of advertising.

Referrals can be encouraged by:

* offering existing clients incentives to introduce new clients to use your service
* establishing links with other professionals by making yourself and what you do known to them.

Public relations

This is a way for aromatherapists to get their name in the public eye without actually paying for advertising.

There is a variety of ways in which it can be done.

1   Offering a free talk and demonstration to a particular client group in the community is an ideal way of marketing aromatherapy and helping to get your name and reputation established.

   Public interest in complementary therapies is increasing all the time and there are many groups that meet regularly who may be keen to hear from you (a list of contact names, addresses and phone numbers may be obtained from your local library).

2   Sending information or news concerning your business to editors of newspapers or magazines in the form of a news article. Every day editors and journalists are looking for stories and information to fill their newspapers or magazines.

   An important consideration when sending information to journalists is only to send information that is truly of interest to the community and their readers.

3   Donating your time, money or products to a local worthwhile charity. There are many charitable organisations that rely on donations each year to survive. An event linked to funding or sponsoring a charity would be a newsworthy article, as well as helping to meet the needs of the community.

4   Getting a regular or one-off slot on the local radio.

5   Compiling a press release, which may be sent to local and national newspapers and magazines. When compiling a press release the following guidelines may help to increase your chance of publication:

* think of an original, interesting, thought-provoking or even humorous headline
* avoid trying to sell your service
* it should be newsworthy and of interest to the journalists and their readers
* address the information directly to a named editor or journalist, preferably one with whom you have already established contact
* ensure that it is laid out clearly (preferably double-lined spaced) and is no longer than two pages
* always include a contact name, address and telephone number.

> ## Key Note
>
> **Editorials in the newspapers and magazines are seen to be credible and true as readers place a considerable amount of trust in the objectivity of journalists.**
>
> **It is therefore worth getting to know editors and journalists and being persistent, as the articles they write tend to hold a lot of weight with readers.**

Indirect approach to marketing and promotion

There are several other methods of advertising or marketing that may be used in order to reach the potential clients you cannot reach in person and these include:

* newspaper advertising
* specialist magazines
* national directories
* mailshots
* leaflets and promotional material
* the internet
* cross merchandising promotional literature

Advertising strategies usually involve a mix of different media and should be scheduled over a period of time for maximum effects. Isolated advertisements rarely sustain enough interest.

Advertising is about getting your message across. Important considerations when considering an advertisement are:

* What do you want to say to potential clients?
* Who is your target audience?
* How will you communicate to them what you want to say?

It is essential to follow the tried and tested AIDA formula when considering your publicity:

A – attracting **attention** – this can be created by an appropriate eye-catching heading

I – generating **interest** – this can be created by stating what is on offer

D – creating **desire** – this can be created by stating why what you have to offer is needed and getting potential clients to believe in the benefits

A – motivating **action** – this can be created by offering the reader an incentive (special offer)

Good advertisements are usually targeted to the right audience, accurate and not misleading, catchy, concise and memorable. Effective adverts must have a good headline (select a major benefit for this) to have immediate impact.

A good headline will:

* attract readers' attention
* compel the person to read further
* improve response
* express the most important benefits.

A good advert should be easy to read and be written to:

* touch people's emotions
* be informative
* promote the service
* raise awareness
* motivate the reader to act.

When designing adverts, ask yourself what adverts you responded to and why.

> **Key Note**
>
> **Words that tend to sell in adverts include:**
>
> **You, New, Results, Health, Free, Complementary, Benefits, Now, Yes.**

Local papers
There are two types of advertisements in newspapers and these are display advertisements and business classified.

Display advertising is more expensive and could appear anywhere in the paper, unless you have paid to have a particular space such as the front or back page, or the television page, which could prove very expensive.

It is always a gamble when relying on display advertising as it may be largely dependent on the following:

* the day of the week the paper is printed
* the time of year
* the page the advert appears on
* the layout of the advert in relation to the other advertisers.

An important point to consider with display advertising is that people buy papers for many reasons other than to read adverts (reading news, announcements and events, crosswords, horoscope). It is therefore important to consider how your advert is going to grab their attention, bearing in mind that newspapers have a short life span, and the AIDA principle.

It is also useful to consider that the person reading the news and features may come across your display advert and may not be thinking about a massage until he or she sees your advert, or they may not be ready to have a massage for some time. In fact it may take many exposures to your advert before this person feels you are sufficiently familiar to give you a try. It is important, therefore, that adverts are repeated regularly in the same way in order to create familiarity. It can also help to have a picture of yourself in the advert as it will be more eye-catching and will help the potential client to feel they know you.

It is important to remember when writing adverts that you are speaking directly to your potential clients and the reader will be initially attracted by your headline message, rather than the name of your business.

It is often helpful to give the reader a cause to reply now, such as a deadline on a special offer, as this motivates action.

When you have designed an advert, it is often helpful to ask friends and colleagues to cast an eye over the design and the wording for critical review. Often another person will spot something you have missed.

Display advertising is usually more effective when it is combined with some editorial. Often papers run special features on health-related matters and it may be more appropriate to consider a display advert within a feature as it draws the reader's attention to a more focused subject.

Classified advertising is more cost effective than display advertising as it is more targeted to the service to be provided. The disadvantage with classified is that there may not always be an appropriate section for aromatherapy and advertising will need to be placed frequently in order to make it effective.

Specialist magazines

These are usually targeted at a specific audience and those related to health are normally of most interest to a holistic therapist. The main drawback is that they are national and whether the advertising will be effective will depend on the readership and the location of the therapist.

> ### Key Note
> **Check the readership profile, circulation radius and readership numbers before committing to advertising in magazines.**

Promotional material

When writing and designing promotional material the key to success is to write it as if you know the client personally. Choose words carefully so that they strike a chord with the client. Remember that many clients reading promotional material may not know they are looking for your service until they see it.

It is also important to ensure that any marketing material reflects the image you wish to portray and that it appeals to the target market. Promotional materials such as leaflets, brochures and posters are the means by

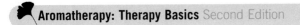

which clients will decide whether to contact you for an appointment. They must be attractive enough to make people want to read them and wording should be positive, direct and, above all, personal. Brochures and posters with a question and answer format can help clients to overcome their objections and visual aids can help to attract attention.

It is also important to use positive language and turn a negative statement (such as a client's problem) into a positive one (how your treatment is going to help them). Including testimonials from satisfied clients (with their permission) can also help to build credibility and break down barriers.

Mailshots

Mailshots can be a worthwhile exercise but require a degree of planning and thought. It is far more effective to target a specific group when designing a mailshot, as the main theme is to address the needs of all the respondents.

You may choose to target self-help groups with a common need of relaxation or to write to the Occupational Health Advisor at local companies offering to give free talks and demonstrations as part of their stress management programme.

The letter should be sent on headed note paper and be brief and concise. The focus should be on the respondent's needs, although it is helpful to send background information on yourself together with information on aromatherapy.

Mailshots usually have a success or response rate of around 2 per cent, although this may be increased to 5 per cent by follow-up phone calls.

Key Note

If writing to companies, it is worth offering the incentive of corporate membership as a promotion to motivate more clients to use your service. Each employee may be issued with a corporate membership card, which entitles them to a certain percentage of discount.

When sending a mailshot, it is important to consider the day it is mailed out as this could have a significant effect on the result.

If you are sending a mailshot to clients' homes, aim for it to arrive on a Friday or Saturday ready for the weekend when they may have more time to consider what you are offering.

If you are sending a mailshot to companies, aim to send the information to arrive on a Tuesday or Wednesday and not a Friday or Monday.

Publications and directories

Advertising in national publications and directories such as *Yellow Pages* can be an effective way of promoting your business, as it is targeted to a specific skill area by virtue of the fact it is classified by therapy type. It is also a long-term form of advertising and can prove to be cost effective as it is a yearly publication.

Aromatherapists should also consider their geographical location and, if they are situated between two counties, it may be advisable to take an advert in more than one directory.

If there are several aromatherapists advertising under the same category then it is important to consider your USP (unique selling point) and stress this in order to give a point of difference from competitors.

Internet

Some aromatherapists are now taking advantage of a web page or site on the internet as a means of advertising their treatments. An attractively designed web page including a treatment menu and a photograph of the therapist may enhance contact from any interested parties.

It is certainly worth considering a web page as a potential source of enquiries and contact, as it is a very cost effective and immediate form of marketing. However, it is also important to remember that not every potential client will have access to the internet and may prefer the more traditional means of contact.

Cross-merchandising promotional literature

Consider other local businesses that cater to clientele similar to yours (such as osteopaths, chiropractors, physiotherapists, health food shops and clinics etc.) and which may be in a position to influence clients to try aromatherapy. Exchange promotional literature and brochures with them; this will give each party additional exposure to the type of clients they wish to attract.

When approaching such businesses with a view to cross merchandising, it is important to establish a friendly, approachable and co-operative working relationship, as this will enhance the success of the promotion on both sides.

Encouraging client retention

The first goal of marketing is to encourage potential clients to try out your services, the next goal is to encourage them to come back again. There are four main ways of fostering repeat business:

* creating an understanding of the benefits of the treatments you provide to clients by encouraging them to book regular treatments

* awarding loyalty bonuses and reward schemes (such as those offered by major supermarket chains)

* staying in touch with your clients and informing them of special offers and any new treatments you may have added to your treatment menu and how they can benefit them

* inviting clients to attend talks and events you may be holding.

Creative marketing opportunities

Other creative marketing opportunities could be to offer gift certificates linked to promotions at specific times of the year such as Christmas, Valentine's Day, birthdays, Mother's Day or Father's Day or for other occasions such as exam successes, etc.

Specially packaged courses of treatments often attract interest as they are designed specifically to address the needs of the respondents.

Professional Ethics

Professional ethics reflect the professional standards and moral principles that govern an aromatherapist's course of action and behaviour. All professional aromatherapy associations publish their own code of ethics that their members are required to follow.

Typical guidelines relating to a code of ethics for aromatherapists are as follows:

* Acknowledge contra-indications for aromatherapy, and refer to the appropriate health professional before any treatment is given.

* Accurately inform clients, members of the public and other health-care professionals of the scope and limitations of aromatherapy.

* Have commitment to the industry in providing the highest quality of service to clients at all times.

* Represent the industry honestly by only providing services in which they are qualified to practise.

* Have respect for the religious, spiritual, social or political views of the client, irrespective of creed, race, colour or sex.

* Never discriminate against other clients, therapists or other health-care professionals.

* Act in a co-operative manner with other health-care professionals and refer cases that are out of the therapy field in which they practise.

* Always present a professional image by practising the highest standards of personal and salon/clinic hygiene.

* Conduct themselves in a professional manner at all times, with honesty and integrity.

* Be courteous to clients and treat them with dignity and respect.

* Keep accurate, up-to-date records of client treatment, including advice given and the outcome/s.

* Safeguard the confidentiality of all client information, unless disclosure is required by law. If liaison is required with a health-care professional, the client's written permission must be sought.

* Provide treatment only when there is reasonable expectation that it will be advantageous to the client.

* Ensure that their working premises comply with all current health, safety and hygiene legislation.

* Never give unqualified advice or claim to cure.

* Never diagnose a medical condition or injury, or prescribe and/or advise the use or disuse of medication.

* Maintain and improve professional development through continuing education and personal development.

* Never abuse the client–therapist relationship.

* Explain the treatment accurately to the client and discuss the fees involved with the client before any treatment commences.

* Ensure that any advertising is accurate, and reflects the professionalism of the industry and that it does not contravene any consumer legislation.

* Be adequately insured to practise the therapy or therapies in which they are qualified.

Setting professional boundaries

In order to have a healthy and professional relationship with clients there should be a balance between care and compassion for the client and keeping a distance from any personal involvement.

The setting of boundaries can provide the foundation upon which an aromatherapist can build a professional relationship with a client. A therapeutic relationship should always involve distance between an aromatherapist and a client, in order to make it safe for both parties. Clients need to be given space to facilitate healing in a therapeutic relationship, and therefore aromatherapists need to keep a healthy distance from a client and their problems.

There is always a risk of transference in a client–therapist relationship, in which a client begins to personalise the professional relationship and thus steps over the professional boundary. There is also a risk of counter-transference when a therapist has difficulty in maintaining a professional distance from the client's problems and begins to step into a friend/counsellor role.

If either of these situations occurs, it is important for a therapist to realise how potentially damaging this can be for a client and how it detracts from their healing process.

Professional Associations

Becoming a member of a professional association helps to give you an identity as a professional and has many other benefits, including:

* a badge and certificate to display to the public, which reflects the trademark of a professional

* professional indemnity insurance at a very reasonable rate, which is negotiated by your professional association

* regular magazines and newsletters, which keep you up to date with the latest information on the industry

* an advisory service

* regular meetings and seminars to meet other colleagues and update your knowledge.

Insurance

Insurance is a necessity in business as it helps to protect your assets. Listed below are different types of insurance:

* **Professional indemnity**   this protects you in the event of a claim arising from malpractice.

* **Public liability**   this protects you in the case of a client or member of the public becoming injured on your premises. The cover may also include damage to a client's property if home visiting.

* **Employer's liability**   this is a legal requirement if you employ staff. It protects an employer against any claims brought about by an employee who may get injured on the premises. A certificate of employer's liability must be displayed in the clinic.

* **Product liability**   this type of insurance protects you against claims arising from products used. In the case of aromatherapy, if you are making up blends for clients' self-use, it is essential for you to have 'selling-on liability'.

* **Buildings insurance**   this protects the building against damage such as fire, explosion, flood or storm damage, accidental damage etc. If you are working from home, review your household policy concerning the liability of operating a business from home. If you are renting, it will usually be the landlord's responsibility to insure the building against the perils listed above. Ask for a copy of the policy to check that it is current.

* **Contents insurance**   this protects the stock, equipment and fittings in your clinic against damage or loss. This cover may also be extended to include equipment and stock if home visiting.

* **Personal accident insurance**   this protects you against loss of income in the event of an accident preventing you from working. Policies of this nature have certain exclusions and restrictions, and advice should be sought from your professional association or through a broker to ensure that you obtain the best policy.

Legal Requirements

An important part of being an aromatherapist and running a clinic is understanding and following health, safety and hygiene regulations to develop safe working practices.

In order to ensure a healthy, safe and secure working environment for yourself, clients and colleagues, it is essential for the aromatherapist to be familiar with the implications of the following legislation and information:

1 **The Industry Code of Practice for Hygiene in Beauty Salons and Clinics**

(published by Vocational Training Charitable Trust). This specifies correct hygiene precautions in order to avoid cross-infection.

2 Legislation relating to **hygiene** and **safety**, including:

* Local Government Miscellaneous Provisions Act 1982

* Local authority bye-laws

* The Health and Safety At Work Act 1974 (procedures in the event of accidents, spillages, breakages)

* Health & Safety (First Aid) Regulation 1981

* Electricity at Work Regulations 1989

* The Personal Protective Equipment at Work Regulations 1992

* Control of Substances Hazardous to Health (COSHH) 1998

* Manual Handling Operations Regulations 1992

* Reporting of Injuries, Diseases and Dangerous Occurrences Regulations 1985 (RIDDOR)

* Dealing with Spillages, Breakages and Waste in the Workplace

* Safety and Security in the Workplace

* Employers' Liability Act 1969

3 **Consumer protection** legislation, including:

* The Sale of Goods Act 1979/The Supply of Goods and Services Act 1982

* The Sale and Supply of Goods Act 1994

* Consumer Protection Act 1987

* Trade Descriptions Act 1968 (amended 1987)

* Data Protection Act 1984

* Performing Rights Act

Legislation relating to health and safety

Health, safety and hygiene are of paramount importance in the workplace. The Law requires that every place of employment is a healthy and safe place, not only for those employees who work there, but also for clients and other visitors who may enter the workplace.

Failure to comply with legislation may have serious consequences such as:

* claims from injured staff or clients

* loss of trade through bad publicity

* closure of the business.

Local Government (Miscellaneous Provisions) Act 1982; Local authority bye-laws

The primary concern of this Act is with efficient hygienic practice.

Bye-laws vary between local authorities, as does the licensing and inspection system involved. Bye-laws are made by the local authority to ensure:

* the cleanliness of the premises and fittings

* the cleanliness and hygiene of the persons registered, and their assistants

* the sterilisation and disinfection of instruments, materials and equipment used.

Large local authorities may have their own legislation under which similar establishments to beauty salons are licensed. In such cases, the licensing may cover what are termed 'special treatments', and this usually includes massage and the provision of ultra-violet treatments. In some areas saunas are licensed and in others they are not.

It is wise to seek the advice of your local authority Environmental Health Officer regarding local legislation that may affect your business.

In areas where licensing and registration are required, it is important to remember that those working from home or undertaking home visiting are still required to register. Only operators working under medical control (as in a hospital) are specifically excluded from registration.

Note: Local Environmental Officers have the authority to fine or cancel the registration of a business that does not maintain and monitor safe hygienic practices.

Health and Safety at Work Act 1974

The Health and Safety at Work Act provides a comprehensive legal framework to promote and encourage high standards of health and safety in the workplace. The Act covers a range of legislation relating to health and safety and both the employer and employee have responsibilities under it. If there are more than five employees a written Health and Safety Policy is required.

The responsibilities of the employer

* To safeguard as far as possible the health, safety and welfare of themselves, their employees, contractors' employees and members of the public.

* To keep all equipment up to health and safety standards.

* To have safety equipment checked regularly.

* To ensure the environment is free from toxic fumes.

* To ensure that all staff are aware of safety procedures, by providing safety information and training.

* To ensure safe systems of work.

The responsibilities of the employee

✳ To adhere to the workplace rules and regulations concerning safety.

✳ To follow safe working practices and attend training as required.

✳ To take reasonable care to avoid injury to themselves and others.

✳ To co-operate with others in all matters relating to health and safety.

✳ Not to interfere with or wilfully misuse anything provided to protect their health and safety.

> ### Key Note
>
> **The Health and Safety Executive (HSE) has produced a guide to the laws on Health and Safety and it is a requirement that an employer displays a copy of this poster in the workplace.**

Health and Safety (First Aid) Regulation 1981

Under the Health and Safety (First-Aid) Regulations 1981 workplaces must have first-aid provision. The form it should take will depend on various factors including the nature and degree of hazards at work, what medical services are available and the number of employees.

The HSE booklet COP 42 First Aid At Work (ISBN 0 11 885536 0) contains an Approved Code of Practice and guidance notes to help employers meet their obligations.

The number of first aiders needed in the workplace depends primarily on the degree of hazards. If the workplace is considered to be low-hazard (such as a holistic therapy clinic) there should be at least one first aider for every 50 employees.

If there are fewer than 50 employees, there should always be an appointed person present when people are at work if no trained first aider is available.

First aiders must undertake training and obtain qualifications approved by the HSE. At present, first-aid certificates are valid for three years. Refresher courses should be started before a certificate expires, otherwise a full course will need to be taken.

First-aid kits

First-aid kits should only contain items that a first aider has been trained to use. They should always be adequately stocked and should **not** contain medication of any kind.

A general purpose first-aid kit will contain the following items: bandages, plasters, wound dressings, antiseptic cream, quick sling, eye pads, scissors, safety pins and vinyl gloves.

First aiders should record all cases they treat. Each record should include at least the name of the patient, date, place, time and circumstances of the accident and details of the injury, and treatment given.

Fire Precautions Act 1971

This legislation is concerned with fire prevention and adequate means of escape in the event of a fire.

The Act enforces that:

* all premises have fire-fighting equipment that is in good working order
* the equipment is readily available and is suitable for all types of fire
* all staff are familiar with the establishment's evacuation procedures and the use of fire-fighting equipment
* fire escapes are kept free from obstruction and clearly signposted
* smoke alarms are fitted
* fire doors are fitted to help control the spread of fire.

Note: It is a legal requirement for an employer to apply for a fire certificate if the business employs 20 or more staff.

It is important for all establishments to have set procedures in the event of a fire and that all staff are aware of them.

Fire extinguishers

There are different fire extinguishers designed to deal with different types of fire. Since 1997, all new fire extinguishers must be coloured red, but they all have different symbols and colour codes to show what type of fire they should be used for.

The main types of fire extinguishers are as follows, with their respective colour code:

* Water (red)
* CO_2 (black)
* Dry Powder (blue)
* Foam (cream).

The above fire extinguishers are colour coded in order to allow quick and easy identification and to avoid using the wrong type and put yourself and others in danger.

The main body colour of the extinguisher has changed over the past few years (any new extinguisher purchased or leased will be predominantly red), however the type colours have remained the same.

Note: Any extinguishers that are not the correct colour will be replaced when they become unserviceable.

Water extinguishers are usually colour-coded red. Other types of extinguisher fall into different categories, either:

* the entire body of the extinguisher is coloured in the type colour
* predominantly red with a 5 per cent second colour to indicate the contents of the extinguisher
* predominantly red with a bold coloured block in the relevant colour stating its type.

If you are in any doubt about the type of fire extinguisher to use in the workplace, it is advisable to contact your local Fire Safety Department for advice.

Electricity at Work Regulations 1989

Regulations under this legislation are concerned with safety in connection with the use of electricity.

It is recommended that electrical equipment be checked regularly (at least once a year) by a competent person such as a qualified electrician or the local electricity board. All checks should be listed in a record book, stating the results of the tests and the recommendations and action taken in the case of defects.

In the case of legal action, a record book may serve as important evidence.

The checks that should be made in connection with electrical equipment include checking the fusing, insulation and that there are no loose or frayed wires.

The Personal Protective Equipment at Work Regulations 1992

This legislation requires an employer to:

✳ provide suitable protective clothing and equipment for all employees to ensure safety in the workplace

✳ ensure staff are adequately trained in the use of chemicals and equipment

✳ ensure that equipment is suitable for its purpose and is kept in a good state of repair.

Control of Substances Hazardous to Health (COSHH) 1998

Regulations under this legislation require employers to regulate employees' exposure to hazardous substances, which may cause ill health or injury in the workplace and involves risk assessment.

Risk assessment involves making an itemised list of all the substances used in the workplace or sold to clients that may be hazardous to health. Attention is drawn to any substances that may cause irritation, allergic reactions, burn the skin or give off fumes.

Instructions for handling and disposing of all hazardous substances must be made available to all staff and training provided, if required.

Manufacturers will usually supply information relating to their products and therapists should be able to recognise hazard warning symbols on labels and packaging.

Manual Handling Operations Regulations 1992

This legislation covers musculo-skeletal disorders primarily caused by manual handling and lifting, repetitive strain disorders and unsuitable posture causing back pain.

The regulations under this legislation cover minimising risks from lifting and handling large or heavy objects and require certain measures to be taken such as correct lifting techniques to avoid musculo-skeletal disorders.

Emergency procedures

In the event of an emergency in the workplace (fire, accident etc.) it is important to remain calm and act quickly:

✳ Dial 999 and ask for the relevant service.

✳ Speak clearly giving details of the emergency.

✳ Listen carefully to any instructions you are given.

Reporting of Injuries, Diseases and Dangerous Occurrences Regulations 1985 (RIDDOR)

This legislation requires that all accidents that occur in the workplace, however minor, **must** be entered into an accident register. This is a requirement of the Health and Safety at Work Act.

An accident report form should detail the following information:

* details of the injured person (age, sex, occupation and contact details)
* date and time of the accident
* place where the accident occurred
* a brief description of the accident
* the nature of the injury
* the action taken
* signatures of all parties concerned (preferable).

The regulations under this legislation also require that, if anyone is seriously injured or dies in connection with an accident in the workplace, or if anyone is off work for more than three days as a result of an accident at work, or if a specified occupational disease is certified by a doctor, then the employer must send a report to the Local Authority Environmental Health Department within seven days.

> **Task**
>
> **Check the health and safety regulations in your college/salon/clinic. What is the procedure in the event of a fire or accident?**

Dealing with spillages, breakages and waste in the workplace

When handling a **spillage**:

* wipe up immediately and warn staff and clientele. If the area is still wet, display a sign indicating the potential hazard.

When handling **breakages**:

* clear up immediately
* wrap up sharp items such as glass before placing them into the waste refuse.

When handling **waste**:

* dispose of in a covered bin
* empty the bin daily.

Safety and security in the workplace

The proprietor of a salon or clinic is required by law to ensure adequate security of their business premises. The following steps may be taken to ensure maximum security. This is important not only for peace of mind but also for insurance requirements.

Security recommendations include:

* fitting locks and bolts on doors and windows
* installing a burglar alarm
* fitting security lights
* ensuring there is a minimum number of key holders
* leaving a light on at night, preferably at the front of the premises
* ensuring all windows and doors are checked before leaving the premises.

Money

* Have a safe for short-term storage of money and valuables.
* Always keep the till locked with a minimum number of key holders.
* Never leave money in the till overnight.

Stock

A good stock control system is needed in the workplace in order to monitor the use of consumables and retail products and this should be documented in a stock control book.

Recommendations for safeguarding stock include:

* always keep supplies in a locked cupboard
* issue keys to a limited number of authorised staff only
* have a locked cabinet for display purposes or use a 'dummy stock' to avoid shoplifting.

Personal belongings

It is not possible for aromatherapists to take responsibility for a client's personal belongings when they attend for treatments. It is important for clients to be aware of this by displaying a disclaimer sign in a reception area.

When clients are removing jewellery, it is important for valuable items to be kept in a safe place for the duration of the treatment. In order to minimise risks, it is advisable to recommend that clients keep a minimum amount of money and valuables on them.

Staff should be vigilant over their own property as well as that of clients and keep handbags and other items of value in a safe place.

Employers' Liability Act 1969

This legislation requires the employer to provide insurance cover against claims for injury or illness as a result of negligence by the employer or other employees.

A certificate of Employers' Liability insurance must be displayed in the workplace.

Consumer legislation

It is important for therapists to be aware of the implications of consumer legislation in the unfortunate event of having to deal with a client seeking compensation for products or services received.

Clients have a right to expect quality in the service they receive, the products used on them during a treatment and products sold to them for home use.

Consumer legislation is designed to protect any person who buys goods or services to ensure that:

* the goods are of merchantable quality

* the goods are not faulty

* there is an accurate description of the good or service.

The Sale of Goods Act 1979/The Supply of Goods and Services Act 1982

As consumers of products and services, clients have rights under the Sale of Goods Act 1979 and the Supply of Goods and Services Act 1982. This legislation identifies the contract of sale, which takes place between the retailer (the clinic/salon) and the consumer (the client).

The Sale of Goods Act 1979 was the first of the laws and covers rights including the goods being accurately described without misleading the consumer.

The Supply of Goods and Services Act 1982 covers rights relating to the standards of service, in that goods and services provided should be of reasonable merchantable quality, described accurately, and be fit for their intended purpose.

The Act also requires that the service provided to a consumer should be carried out with reasonable skill and care, within a reasonable time and for a reasonable cost.

The Sale and Supply of Goods Act 1994

This legislation amends the previous Acts and has introduced guidelines on defining the quality of goods.

Consumer Protection Act 1987

This Act provides the consumer with protection when buying goods or services to ensure that products are safe for use on the client during the treatment, or are safe to be sold as a retail product.

The Act provides the same rights to anyone injured by a defective product, whether the product was sold to them or not.

The Act also covers giving misleading price indications about goods, services or facilities. The term 'price indication' also includes price comparisons. To be misleading includes any wrongful indications about conditions attached to a price, about what you expect to happen to a price in the future and what you say in price comparisons.

It is essential to understand the implications of this legislation, including the promotion of special offers, as an offence could result in legal proceedings.

Trade Descriptions Act 1968 (amended 1987)

This Act prohibits the use of false descriptions or to sell or offer the sale of goods that have been described falsely. It covers advertisements such as oral descriptions, display cards and applies to quality and quantity as well as fitness for purpose and price.

It is important to understand its provision, where the description is given by another person and repeated. Thus to repeat a manufacturer's claim is to be equally liable.

Data Protection Act 1984

This legislation protects clients' personal information being stored on a computer.

If client records are stored on computer, the establishment must be registered under this Act.

The Data Protection Act operates to ensure that the information stored is used only for the purposes for which it was given.

Businesses should therefore ensure that they:

* only hold information that is relevant
* allow individuals access to the information held on them
* prevent unauthorised access to the information.

Performing Rights Act

If a therapist is using relaxation music when carrying out aromatherapy treatments in the workplace it may be necessary to obtain a licence from Phonographic Performance Ltd (PPL) or the Performing Rights Society (PRS), an organisation that collects licence payments as royalties on behalf of performers and record companies whose music is protected under the Copyright Designs and Patent Act 1998.

When seeking to play music in treatment premises it is important to check whether the music is copyright free, in which case no licence fee is due, or whether it is protected under this legislation.

Self-assessment Questions

1. What are the responsibilities of an employer under the Health and Safety at Work Act 1974?

----

2. State four requirements of the Fire Precautions Act 1971.

----

3. Explain what is meant by the legislation entitled COSHH.

----

4. What is the importance of adhering to consumer legislation as a practising aromatherapist?

----

5. State five important types of insurance requirements when practising as an aromatherapist.

----

6. Why are professional ethics important to a practising aromatherapist?

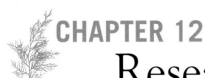

CHAPTER 12
Research in Aromatherapy

> *Owing to the increased public and professional interest in aromatherapy, there is a growing need for aromatherapists to justify their work in terms of its efficacy, cost-effectiveness and safety.*
>
> *If aromatherapy is to gain recognition, it is necessary for research to be carried out in order that benefits may be assessed critically and objectively.*
>
> *This chapter gives a general overview as to how aromatherapists may approach research in order to extend their professional development.*

Objectives

By the end of this chapter you will be able to relate the following knowledge to your work as an aromatherapist:

* the advantages and disadvantages of research
* the stages involved in developing a research proposal
* seeking possible sources of funding
* how to access research data on aromatherapy.

Research can be stimulating, challenging and rewarding but it should be remembered that it is a very time-consuming process that requires both time and commitment.

The advantages for the aromatherapist are that it adds credibility to the aromatherapy professional and is an excellent learning tool in aiding professional development.

Practical disadvantages are that a chosen project may require significant funding and/or involve a considerable amount of time. It is always possible that after the research has been carried out it may prove that initial expectations are unconfirmed.

Getting Started

The first decision to make is to identify clearly an area of aromatherapy of interest and define the objectives of the project. It is useful to read research projects that have already been undertaken, which will give you ideas for ways of approaching research based on the methodology and results of others. It will also help you to ascertain whether anybody else has attempted research in your chosen area of interest, along with the positive and negative aspects of the research.

University libraries are a good source of reference for reading material for ideas along with the Research Council for Complementary Medicine (RCCM) (see below) and professional journals such as the *International Journal of Aromatherapy* (see Resource section).

The RCCM and its Centralised Information Service for Complementary Medicine (CISCOM) can provide help with literature searches and guidance regarding research methodology. The RCCM now provides a service that facilitates an evidence-based approach to complementary and integrative medicine by using specialist skills and drawing on the CISCOM database. The database contains around 70,000 research references with some 1064 on aromatherapy. A CISCOM Search Request is available on payment of £20 covering from one to 50 references and a form is available from the RCCM, Suite 5, 1 Harley Street, London W1G 9QD or by e-mail to **info@rccm.org.uk** Their website address is: **www.rccm.org.uk**

Self-help groups in an area of chosen interest are another source of reference and access to these may be through GP surgeries/health clinics, hospitals and the internet. Local branches are often advertised in local newspapers.

Aromatherapy Database – research into the psychophysiological properties of essential oils and their components, 800 references and abstracts from published research papers sourced from over 200 professional journals worldwide. Contact: EORC, 'Au village', 83840 La Martre, Provence, France, Tel/Fax: (33) 494 84 29 93, www.essentialorc.com.

Turning the Research Idea into a Proposal

Once you have read about your chosen area sufficiently, the next stage is to turn the research idea into a research proposal.

A research proposal involves a detailed written plan of the research you intend to conduct, which needs to be specific and measurable.

A research proposal is important as it:

* helps to clarify the main objectives of the proposal
* demonstrates your commitment
* is a means of communicating the objectives to other partners you want to involve in the research
* is a necessary requirement for obtaining funding and support to implement the project.

A general outline for a research proposal is as follows:

* Title
* A summary of your qualifications and experience (evidence that you are a suitable person to conduct the proposed research)
* Summary of objectives
* Literature review
* Planned methodology for collecting data
* Budget for the proposal
* Proposed time frame for its completion.

It is at this stage that contact should be made with possible partners for the research, ideally those whose daily work involves research design and implementation. Possible sources of contact are:

* University departments (especially if they run courses in complementary health) that already publish research in related subjects and may be able to put you in touch with a researcher who can advise or assist in the development of research methodology

* NHS trusts/primary care groups or GP practices

* Royal College of Nursing, Complementary Therapies Special Interest Group, 20 Cavendish Square, London WIM 0AB (www.rcn.org.uk)

* Clinicians or scientists (may be hospital or university based)

* Medical Ethics Committees attached to local health authorities

* Schools of Aromatherapy (it is helpful to select one that is linked to a University)

* Aromatherapy associations

* Practitioners of aromatherapy or another field of complementary therapy

* Essential Oil Resource Consultants (see useful addresses at the back of this book).

It is important to gain expert advice when undertaking research, so that your project will be taken seriously. You need to consider fully not only how the research will be carried out, but most importantly how it will be analysed and presented. Expert advice is therefore essential in the methodology, design and analysis stages as research needs to be carried out and presented in such a way that it can stand up to scientific scrutiny.

Experienced researchers have the necessary expertise and resources that fledgling researchers need so it is advisable to seek their help as much as possible.

Seeking Funding

Another important consideration is how the project will be funded. There are a number of organisations that offer support, advice and sponsorship to individuals with sound research proposals.

The AOC has a list of bodies that may provide funding for research projects. When contacting possible sponsors it is important to be clear and specific in your proposal and to develop your application to meet their criteria.

The RCCM also encourages and sponsors research into complementary medicine.

Once you have gained the resources and necessary support to conduct the research it is important to stay focused, as research is very time consuming and at times can be very challenging. Seeing a research project through to the end can have enormous rewards as there is ultimately the satisfaction of having the research published, and the opportunity to make a difference by influencing practice in the industry.

Task

Research an area of aromatherapy that interests you and report your findings, using the guidelines given in this chapter.

You may wish to consider the following:

* Is aromatherapy currently being used locally, or nationally in your chosen aspect of research, and if so where and how?

* How long has aromatherapy been used in this field?

* How effective has aromatherapy been and how has this been measured?

* Are there any particular essential oils or forms of treatment found to be most effective?

* If aromatherapy has not been used in your chosen area of research, is there a possible business practice opportunity?

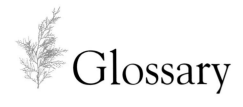

Glossary

Analgesic: relieves pain

Antidepressant: uplifting, counteracting melancholy, alleviates depression

Anti-haemorrhagic: prevents or combats bleeding

Anti-inflammatory: alleviates inflammation

Anti-microbial: destroys or resists pathogenic micro-organisms

Anti-rheumatic: helps relieve and prevent rheumatism

Antiseptic: destroys and prevents the development of microbes

Antispasmodic: relieves cramp, prevents or eases spasms or convulsions

Antiviral: substance that inhibits the growth of a virus

Aperitif: stimulates the appetite

Aphrodisiac: increases or stimulates sexual desire

Astringent: contracts bodily tissues, helps to control infection

Bactericidal: an agent that destroys bacteria

Carminative: relieves flatulence (wind) by expelling gas from the intestines

Cephalic: stimulates and clears the mind

Cytophylactic: encourages cell regeneration

Decongestant: releases nasal mucus

Deodorant: reduces odour

Depurative: helps combat impurities, detoxifying

Detoxifying/ detoxicant: helps cleanse the body of impurities

Diuretic: stimulates the secretion of urine

Emmenagogue: induces or assists menstruation

Expectorant: aids the removal of catarrh

Febrifuge: combats fever

Fungicidal: kills or inhibits the growth of yeasts, moulds etc.

Haemostatic: arrests bleeding/haemorrhage

Hepatic: tonic to the liver, aids functioning of liver

Hypertensive: increases blood pressure

Hypotensive: lowers blood pressure

Hormonal: balances or regulates the body's hormonal secretion

Immunostimulant: stimulates the body's own natural defence system

Insecticidal: repels insects

Laxative: promotes elimination of the bowels

Nervine: strengthens the nervous system

Parasiticidal: destroys and prevents parasites

Parturient: aids childbirth

Relaxant: soothes, induces relaxation, relieves strain or tension

Rubefacient: increases local circulation, creates erythema, warming

Sedative: produces a calming effect

Stimulant: has a rousing, uplifting effect on the mind and body

Stomachic: digestive aid and tonic, improves appetite

Tonic: strengthens and enlivens the whole or specific parts of the body

Uterine: tonic to the uterus

Vasodilator: an agent that dilates the blood vessels

Vasoconstrictor: an agent that causes narrowing of the blood vessels

Vulnerary: helps heal wounds and sores

Bibliography

Berwick, Ann (1994) *Holistic Aromatherapy*, Llewellyn Publication

Bettelheim & March (1990) *Introduction to Organic Biochemistry*

Davis, Patricia (1995) *Aromatherapy, an A–Z*, C.W. Daniel Company Ltd

Harris, Rhiannon (1999) *Becoming an Aromatherapist*, How to Books

Lawless, Julia (1994) *Aromatherapy and the Mind*, Thorsons

Lawless, Julia (1995) *The Illustrated Encyclopaedia of Essential Oils*, Elements Books

Mojay, Gabriel (1996) *Aromatherapy for Healing the Spirit*, Gaia Books Ltd

Price, Shirley (1993) *Shirley Price's Aromatherapy Workbook*, Thorsons

Price, Shirley and Len (1995) *Aromatherapy for Health Professionals*, Churchill Livingstone

Rosser, Mo (1996) *Body Massage Therapy Basics*, Hodder & Stoughton

Skoog, West & Holler (1992) *Fundamentals of Analytical Chemistry*

Tisserand, Robert (1991) *The Art of Aromatherapy*, C.W. Daniel Company Ltd

Tisserand, Robert and Balacs, Tony (1995) *Essential Oil Safety, A Guide for Health Professionals*, Churchill Livingstone

Valnet, Dr Jean (1991) *The Practice of Aromatherapy*, C.W. Daniel Company Ltd

Vickers, Andrew (1996) *Massage and Aromatherapy: A Guide for Health Professionals*, Chapman & Hall

Watt, Martin (1994) *Plant Aromatics*, private publication

Wildwood, Chrissie (1996) *The Bloomsbury Encyclopaedia of Aromatherapy*, Bloomsbury

Williams, David G. (1996) *The Chemistry of Essential Oils*, Micelle Press

Worwood, Valerie Ann (1995) *The Fragrant Mind*, Bantam Books

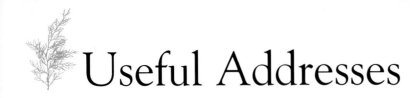

Useful Addresses

Essential Oils

Butterbur & Sage
7 Tessa Road
Reading
Berkshire
RG1 8HH
Tel: 0118 950 5100
www.butterburandsage.com

Natural Touch
Hilton House
Mayles Lane
Wickham
Hants
PO17 5ND
01329 833220
www.naturaltoucharomatherapy.com

Fragrant Earth
Orchard Court
Magdalene Street
Glastonbury
Somerset
BA6 9WE
Tel: 01458 831216
www.fragrant-earth.com

Professional Journals

Aroma Publications (produce a magazine called *Aromatica*)
PO Box 22771
London
N22 6ZN

Aromatherapy Today
Alembic Publishing
36 Cotham Hill
Bristol
BS6 6LA
Tel: 0117 908 7770

International Journal of Aromatherapy
Elsevier Science
32 Jamestown Rd
London
NW1 7BY
(it is possible to subscribe online at Amazon.com)

Aromatic Thymes
18–4 E Dundee Road
Suite 200
Barrington
IL 60010
USA
Tel: (847) 304–0975
Email: aromatic@interaccess.com

Professional Associations

The Federation of Holistic Therapists
3rd Floor
Eastleigh House
Eastleigh
Hampshire
SO50 9FD
Tel: 02380 684500
www.fht.org.uk

The International Federation of Professional Aromatherapists (IFPA) (incorporating the IFA, ISPA and the RQA)
82 Ashby Rd
Hinckley
Leics
LE10 1SN
Tel: 01455 637987
Email: admin@ifparoma.org

The International Guild of Professional Practitioners (incorporating the Guild of Complementary Practitioners and ITEC Professionals)
4 Heathfield Terrace
Chiswick
London
W4 4JE
Tel: 020 8994 7856
Email: professionals@itecworld.co.uk
www.igpp.co.uk

General

Aromatherapy Organisations Council (AOC)
PO Box 19834
London
SE25 6WF
www.aoc.uk.net

Aromatherapy Trade Council (ATC)
PO Box 387
Ipswich
Suffolk
IP2 9AN
Tel/Fax: 01473 603630
E.mail: info@a-t-c.org.uk

Essential Oil Resource Consultants (EORC)
Au Village
83840 La Martre
Provence
France
Tel/Fax: (33) 494 84 29 93
essentialorc@aol.com

Index